Praise for
MAXIMUM STRENGTh

"Eric Cressey is equal parts academic scholar and in-the-trenches veteran. It's hard enough to find a fitness expert who exhibits one of these qualities, let alone a man who exemplifies both. . . . Cressey is a complete professional."

—SEAN HYSON, Fitness Editor, *Men's Fitness*, *Sly*, and *Muscle & Fitness* magazines

"*Maximum Strength* is a guide for those who truly want to make meaningful changes to their bodies. Eric Cressey has created a program that will challenge any individual to push themselves to levels they have never been before. In the years that I have known Eric, his goal to help people achieve maximum performance and get the most out of their bodies has never wavered."

—MICHAEL IRR, BS, CSCS, Assistant Strength Coach, Chicago Bulls

"Eric Cressey is one of the sharpest minds in the field of performance enhancement today. His ability to apply his knowledge in an efficient, progressive, and comprehensive manner is outstanding. He continues to be a fundamental resource for me in this profession."

—CHRIS WEST, MS, CSCS, ATC, Associate Head Coach,
Strength and Conditioning, University of Connecticut

"Eric Cressey has outdone himself with *Maximum Strength*. The average gym-goer has been needlessly pumping away with sets of 8–10 repetitions for years, with no real gains to show for it. Instead, we know that many of these guys would see amazing gains if they'd simply focus on getting stronger first and foremost. *Maximum Strength* has all the tools to play an integral role in someone's long-term success. Do yourself a favor and pick up a copy today. You'll get stronger, feel better, and see some real changes in your body for the first time in a long time."

—MIKE ROBERTSON, www.RobertsonTrainingSystems.com

"I've been involved in the strength-training industry for over 14 years and I can safely say that this is one of the best books on the topic I've come across. Very well laid out, easy to follow, and the sample bonus programs Eric includes are invaluable. It deserves to be on the bookshelf of every athlete, trainer, and coach."

—RYAN LEE, founder, StrengthCoach.com

ERIC CRESSEY, MA, CSCS, renowned strength coach and record-setting powerlifter, is the author of *The Ultimate Off-Season Training Manual* and cocreator of the *Magnificent Mobility* DVD and *Building the Efficient Athlete* DVD set. A regular contributor to *Testosterone Nation, Men's Fitness,* and Elite Fitness Systems, Eric is the owner of Cressey Performance, which features two strength and conditioning facilities in the Greater Boston area. He lives in Framingham, Massachusetts. www.EricCressey.com

MATT FITZGERALD is the author/coauthor of seven books, including *Brain Training for Runners* and *Triathlon Magazine's Complete Triathlon Book.* He writes regularly for such national publications as *Maxim, Men's Fitness, Men's Health, Runner's World, Triathlete,* and *Maximum Fitness* and for Web sites such as www.Active.com and Runner's World Online. A triathlete, runner, and coach, he lives in San Diego, California. www.mattfitzgerald.org

MAXIMUM
STRENGTH

MAXIMUM STRENGTH

GET YOUR STRONGEST BODY IN 16 WEEKS WITH THE ULTIMATE WEIGHT-TRAINING PROGRAM

ERIC CRESSEY, MA, CSCS

MATT FITZGERALD

Da Capo

LIFE
LONG

A Member of the Perseus Books Group

Designed by Pauline Brown

Set in 9.5 point Bell Gothic by the Perseus Books Group

Cataloging-in-Publication data for this book is available from the Library of Congress.

First Da Capo Press edition 2008

ISBN: 978-1-60094-057-6

Published by Da Capo Press

A Member of the Perseus Books Group

www.dacapopress.com

Note: The information in this book is true and complete to the best of our knowledge. This book is intended only as an informative guide for those wishing to know more about health issues. In no way is this book intended to replace, countermand, or conflict with the advice given to you by your own physician. The ultimate decision concerning care should be made between you and your doctor. We strongly recommend you follow his or her advice. Information in this book is general and is offered with no guarantees on the part of the authors or Da Capo Press. The authors and publisher disclaim all liability in connection with the use of this book.

Da Capo Press books are available at special discounts for bulk purchases in the United States by corporations, institutions, and other organizations. For more information, please contact the Special Markets Department at the Perseus Books Group, 2300 Chestnut Street, Suite 200, Philadelphia, PA 19103, or call (800) 255–1514, or e-mail special.markets@perseusbooks.com.

10 09 08 07 06 05 04 03

To my parents,
Susan and George Cressey,
for sticking with me through the thick—
and definitely the thin.

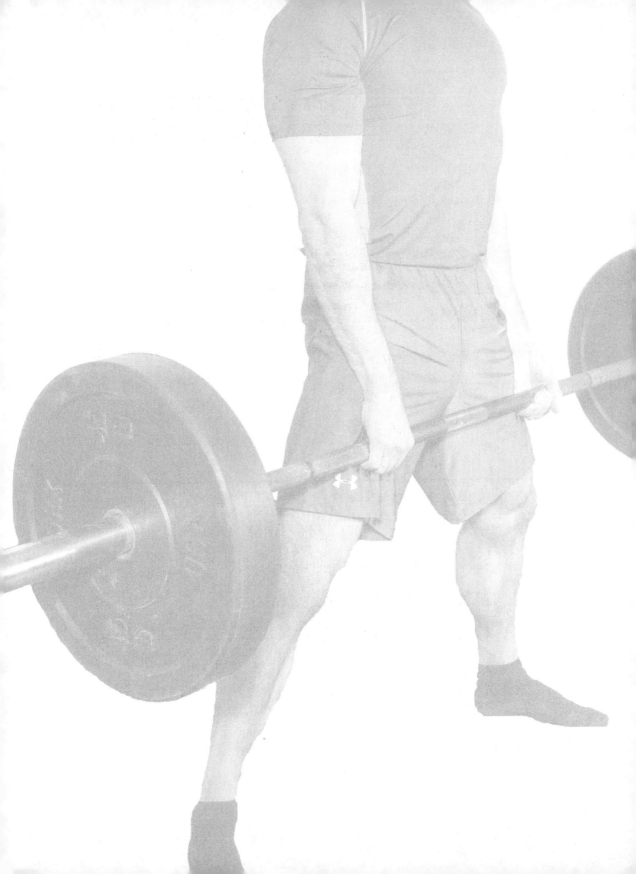

CONTENTS

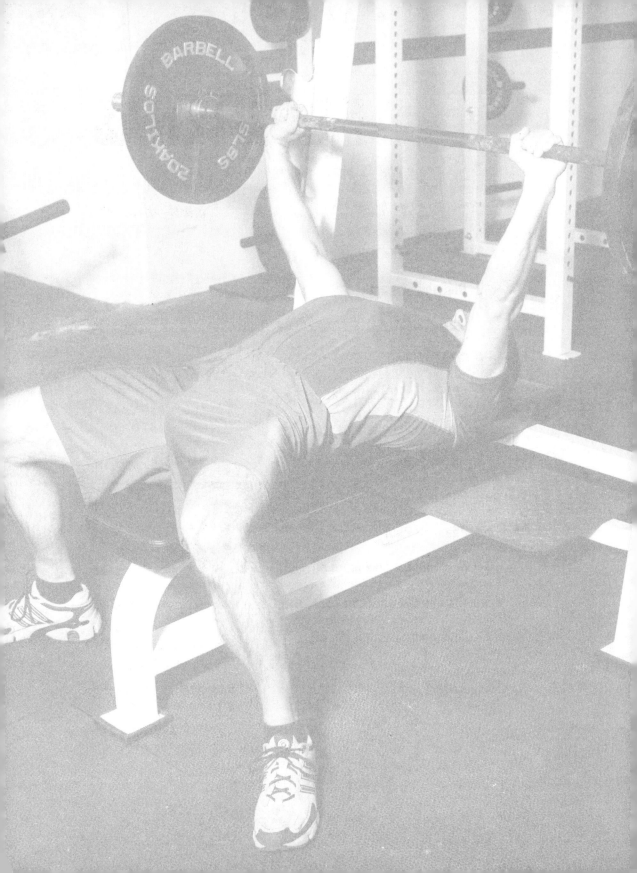

FOREWORD

by John Berardi, PhD

A few years back, when my personal Web site was publishing the work of up-and-coming coaches, trainers, and nutritionists, I received an e-mail from a young Eric Cressey. Eric, a recent university graduate and weightlifting enthusiast, had decided to try his hand at writing and was wondering if I'd be interested in publishing an article he'd recently put together. The article was all about teaching weightlifters how to budget for things like gym memberships, gym equipment, healthy food, and nutritional supplements—and it was pretty good. So I decided to run it. Interestingly, more than 30,000 readers checked out the article. And they loved it.

I had no idea that this type of article would have such an impact. But Eric did. You see, Eric's a true problem solver. By nature he looks for areas that can be improved upon and sets out to make those improvements. Back when he sent me that first article, he recognized a specific problem people were having. And he set out to find a solution. Of course, by nature, he hasn't let up since.

Foreword

Impressively, since that first article, Eric's star has been on the rise. Over the past few years, he has established himself as one of the top exercise and performance specialists in the world, a guy people come to in order to build muscle strength, to boost muscle size, and to improve their fitness. It doesn't hurt that he's earned a master's degree in exercise science from the prestigious University of Connecticut, studying under top strength researchers Dr. William Kraemer, Dr. Carl Maresh, and Dr. Jeff Volek. It probably doesn't hurt either that he's published more than 250 articles on strength training, he's brought to market several books and DVD products in the area of strength training and athletic preparation, and he's personally helped hundreds of athletes and recreational exercisers reach their goals. Nor does it hurt that he's a guy who both talks the talk and walks the walk.

Eric Cressey is one strong SOB. Seriously, how many 165-pound guys do you know who can bench-press over 400 pounds, deadlift over 600 pounds, and squat over 500 pounds? Heck, I'm in the high-performance field and I don't know that many. And Cressey wasn't born strong. Nor did his parents feed baby Cressey massive quantities of spinach while having him pull a plate-loaded red wagon for exercise. In fact, he grew up fairly chubby and unathletic. But with the right plan (and a good amount of heart) he built his strength from the ground up. And you can, too.

Now, I know what you're thinking. Just because a guy can figure out how to get himself strong doesn't mean he knows how to get you strong. And you're right. However, that's where you have to look past Cressey's barrel chest to the results he consistently produces with others—results that you'll be able to read about as you progress through the Maximum Strength Program. For example, check out Chris Paul on page 37. He gained 80 pounds on his box squat, 30 pounds on his bench press, and 50 pounds on his deadlift in just 16 weeks by following the Maximum Strength Program. Also make sure to read about Dan Hibbert on page 37. He also gained 80 pounds on his box squat, 30 pounds on his bench press, and 70 pounds on his deadlift on the same program.

These results are no fluke. The Maximum Strength Program formula is well researched in the science lab and well proven in the real-world "lab" known as the gym. Would you expect anything less from a guy who's learned it in school, who's done it in the real world, and who continues to teach it successfully?

By now it should be obvious that I highly respect Eric Cressey's professional expertise and that I wholeheartedly believe in the power of the Maximum Strength Program. Indeed, I know that if you consistently apply the principles you're about to learn, you'll be turning heads both in and out of the gym. While training, your gym mates will wonder how the heck you're making progress with every single workout—specially when they've been dedicated but stagnant for years! And your nonworkout friends will wonder whether you've been washing your cotton shirts on high heat or you're simply packing too much muscle for your wardrobe. Either way, I'm sure you'll be fine with both sets of observations.

However, one of the best parts about this particular book is that you'll not only learn how to lift for increased muscle strength and size but also learn a host of other valuable lessons—like how to lift pain- and injury-free. That's right; get out your foam rollers, folks, and start doing those mobility drills. The injury prevention segment of the program is worth its weight in gold, as it'll help resolve previous muscle and joint pain as well as help prevent these aches and pains from rearing their ugly heads in the future. My clients and I swear by this book's warm-up methods.

Another huge "value-added" element is the nutrition section. Being a nutrition coach and all, I may be a bit biased—especially as many of the strategies in Chapter 10 are strategies Cressey and his coauthor, Matt Fitzgerald, stole from me. But in all seriousness, if you commit to applying the nutrition suggestions provided in Chapter 10, your weightroom progress will be light years ahead of that of your peers. And on top of it all, you'll have better health and a leaner physique to show for it.

I could go on and on about how great Eric is and how much I like this book. But you probably want to get right down to it. So I'll wrap up here. If you've been looking for the right recipe to get strong—seriously strong—step into the Cressey kitchen. Backed by both science and results, the Maximum Strength Program template Eric and Matt have provided in the coming pages will change the way you view strength training—while changing both the way you look and the way your body performs.

In strength,

John Berardi, PhD, CSCS

Dr. John Berardi is one of North America's most popular and respected authorities on fitness and nutrition. He has made his mark as a leading researcher in the field of exercise and nutritional science, as a widely read author and writer, and as a coach and trainer to thousands of elite athletes and recreational exercisers. Currently Dr. Berardi is the president of Precision Nutrition—a world leader in nutritional programming for active men and women. You can find out more at www.precisionnutrition.com.

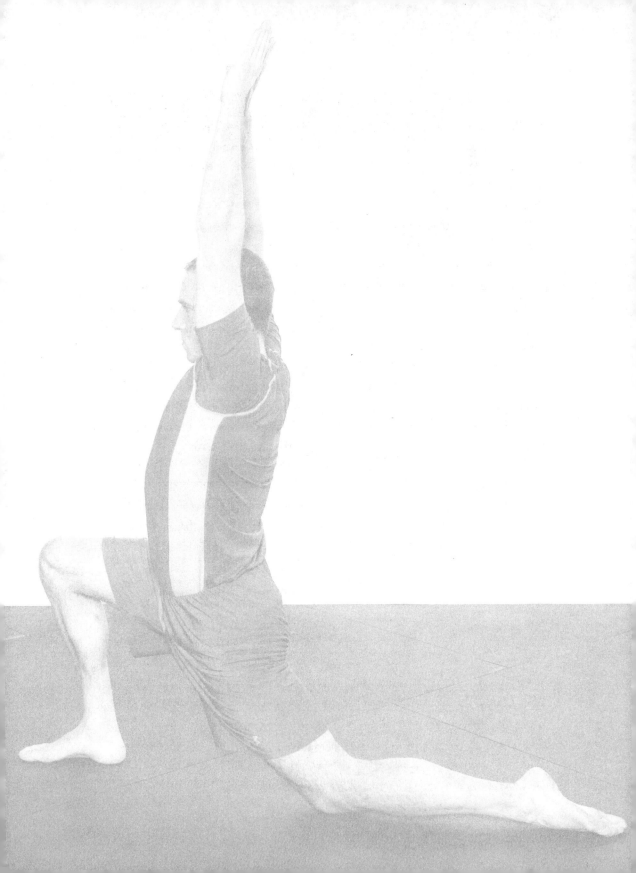

INTRODUCTION

When I was a little boy running around on the school playground, I dreamed of being the strongest man in the world, not the largest man in the world. I liked to imagine all the cool stuff I could do with superstrength, like hit a baseball into the next town and pin bullies to the ground with one arm. The notion of having super size without matching strength held no appeal for me whatsoever. How much fun would it be to merely *look* as if I could hit a baseball into the next town if I actually couldn't? None!

Years later, however, when I got into weightlifting, I was somehow brainwashed into thinking I wanted to be massive instead of mighty. The same thing happens to most American males who choose weightlifting as their primary fitness activity. Somewhere between the playground and the office cubicle they lose their childhood wisdom and trade the dream of being the strongest man in the world for that of being the largest man in the room.

This unfortunate substitution comes with significant consequences. The most effective methods of increasing strength are drastically different from the watered-down bodybuilding methods most guys use to pursue greater mass. Training for maximum strength is much more fun, because your progress is more steady and easy to quantify. It's all about adding weight to the bar instead of squinting into the mirror, trying to see whether your shirt is fitting more tightly than it did four weeks ago. Scientific research has also shown that increasing your strength produces greater benefits in terms of health and real-world performance than merely increasing your muscle size. You really can accomplish much more with strong muscles than big muscles, and strong muscles also do a better job of keeping you lean, preventing degenerative diseases such as diabetes, and even slowing the aging process. Increasing your maximum strength is simply one of the most beneficial things you can do for yourself, whether your main goal is to improve your performance in any sport, enhance your overall health, build self-confidence and improve your sex life, or live to see your 100th birthday.

Fortunately, I rediscovered the superiority of muscle strength to muscle size while studying exercise physiology as a graduate student at the University of Connecticut. Over the next several years I threw myself into learning and creating the most effective methods to develop maximum strength. I now use these methods with a wide range of clients, from professional athletes to grandfathers who just want to get around better, whom I train in my fitness facility in Boston, Massachusetts, and online.

These same methods are also the basis of the 16-week Maximum Strength training program that I will guide you through in this book. In the Maximum Strength Program you will swap the goal of getting bigger for a better goal of getting stronger, and you'll leave behind those tired, old watered-down bodybuilding workouts for the cutting-edge strength-building sessions detailed in the following chapters. As a result you will become stronger than you have ever been. You will also become more functionally sound—familiar sore spots and weak links in your body will vanish—and you will experience improvement in any and all sports you may participate in. You will enjoy your training sessions more than ever before, and your confidence will reach new heights, in part because your physique will inch closer to that perfect 10 rating you've always coveted. Finally, you will shed body fat, and yes, if you are still interested in gaining muscle mass, you will find it easier to do that, too.

How can I be so confident that you will experience such great results? Because I see them every day in my clients. And my first client was me. My entire life changed when I took up powerlifting several years ago. In just eight weeks I went from being an unemployed videogame addict living in my parents' basement to the lead singer of a band with a Billboard Top 10 single.

Not buying it? OK, what really happened when I started powerlifting was that I not only found the sport I was truly born for but I also broke out of a prolonged period of staleness and stagnation in my pursuit of a better body. At the time the opportunity to become a powerlifter came along and rescued me, I was working out with the vague goal of putting on a little muscle mass, just like 99 percent of the other guys with fitness club memberships. My pursuit of a better body was all about appearance, not performance. Consequently, my "routine" was just that: *routine*. I lacked focus and direction and was really just spinning my wheels at the gym. After weeks and weeks of working out using traditional bodybuilding methods, I might put on half a pound of muscle, which is barely even quantifiable and certainly not a very motivating result for so much sweat and effort.

Working out was a part of my lifestyle that I enjoyed, but it no longer had the excitement that it previously had when I was a competitive tennis and soccer player in high school, training to win and seeing myself improve every season. I was involved in varsity strength and conditioning at the University of Connecticut, and each day I looked around and saw that same excitement in the athletes with whom I was working; they were *training* for something, not just "working out." I had to find an outlet for my competitive side—and a pursuit in which I could quantify my progress. Some friends who knew of my frustration suggested I try powerlifting, and boy, am I glad I listened to them!

Two things changed when I started powerlifting: my training methods and my mindset. As you will quickly discover in reading this book and following my Maximum Strength Program, the methods used to train for maximum strength are very different from those used to increase muscle mass. In essence, the difference is bigger movements, heavier weights, and fewer reps. I couldn't believe how quickly my strength improved when I traded my bodybuilding routine for a powerlifting program. In September 2003 I tested my maximum deadlift at 429 pounds. Just over nine months later, I pulled 510 pounds at my first meet, beating the old American Powerlifting Association Connecticut Junior 165-pound-weight-class state record by more than 60 pounds. And the stronger I got, the more everything fell into place. My muscle balance improved, some old aches and pains went away, and I found it easier to gain muscle and lose fat.

That's right: lose fat. At the time I took up powerlifting I was lucky enough to have a DEXA scan done. (A DEXA scanner measures body composition by imaging the inside of the body. It's considered the most accurate body-fat-assessment technology in existence.) I then weighed 171.6 pounds, at a height of 5 feet 8 inches. The scanner reported that I was 14.6 percent body fat, and my bone density was 1.226 g/cm². Conveniently enough, just under one year later, I scored an opportunity to have a second scan done. I knew my body had changed significantly, but I wasn't ready for the astounding results I saw.

After one year of powerlifting (including four meets) my weight had gone up by 3.5 pounds to 175.1 pounds, but I had *dropped 3.7 percent in body fat* to 10.5 percent. (And, by the way, if that number sounds high, be advised that DEXA scan measurements of body fat are usually 3 to 4 percent higher than those produced by other methods, which systematically underestimate body fat percentage.) Meanwhile, my lean body mass had increased 7.9 percent. This change equates to an 11.26-pound increase in lean body mass with a simultaneous drop of 5.46 pounds of body fat on a frame that was already pretty lean. Just as impressively, my bone density had risen 6.2 percent. I had added approximately $^1/_3$ *of a pound of pure bone* to my body!

Even more important to me than these results was the change in mind-set that I experienced after becoming a powerlifter. Powerlifting gave me concrete, meaningful, quantifiable goals to pursue. No longer was I squinting in the mirror, trying to see whether the past month of doing the same old thing had resulted in any visible changes in my physique ("Was that vein always so visible?"). Now I was counting the plates on the bar. Each time the weight increased, I felt rewarded for my hard work and got a shot of motivation to increase the weight even more. My passion for exercise was fully reawakened. Going to the gym was exciting again, and it was all because I had changed my focus from appearance to performance. This shift in mind-set gave my training regimen the focus and direction it had been lacking.

In fact, my entire life aligned itself around my new goals in synergistic ways. For example, instead of merely trying to eat right so I wouldn't get fat, I was now nourishing and fueling my body to get stronger, and this new purpose made it easier to eat even more healthily than I had previously. And to top it all off, women started throwing themselves at me. Well, maybe not, but I did receive a lot more compliments on my physique than I had in a long time!

Now, you don't have to become a competitive powerlifter, as I did, to get all of these benefits. Only a small fraction of my clients are competitive powerlifters, but virtually all of my clients train for and increase their maximum strength and also improve their performance in sports and everyday activities, as well as their appearance, overall health, and self-confidence. I wrote *Maximum Strength* to help out the countless guys who are caught in the same rut I was stuck in a few years ago: the rut of boredom and stagnating results that comes from endlessly pursuing the vague and pointless goal of getting bigger with inefficient, outmoded bodybuilding routines. The way out that worked for me, and that also works for my gym clients and online clients, will work for you, too: training for maximum strength instead of maximum size.

The Maximum Strength Program is a 16-week training program that's divided into four phases lasting four weeks apiece, each with its own training emphasis. The weekly training schedule entails two upper-body strength sessions and two lower-body strength sessions. Optional cardio workouts are also provided to supplement the training program. (I'll cover nutrition and mental training techniques in the book's later chapters.) The program culminates in a four-lift maximum strength test on the final day, which I call "Moving Day," to emphasize the real-world benefits of achieving maximum strength. When you complete the program you will be amazed by the amount of weight you are able to bench-press, squat, deadlift, and chin-up after just 16 weeks of focused training. In the book's final chapter, I will show you how to transform the basic structure of the Maximum Strength Program into an ongoing training approach that will enable you to keep getting stronger for some time to come.

Are you ready to find out just how strong you can be? Then I'm your magic genie, here to grant your wish. The only catch is that you have to bust your ass to get this wish. I just lead the way. So follow me!

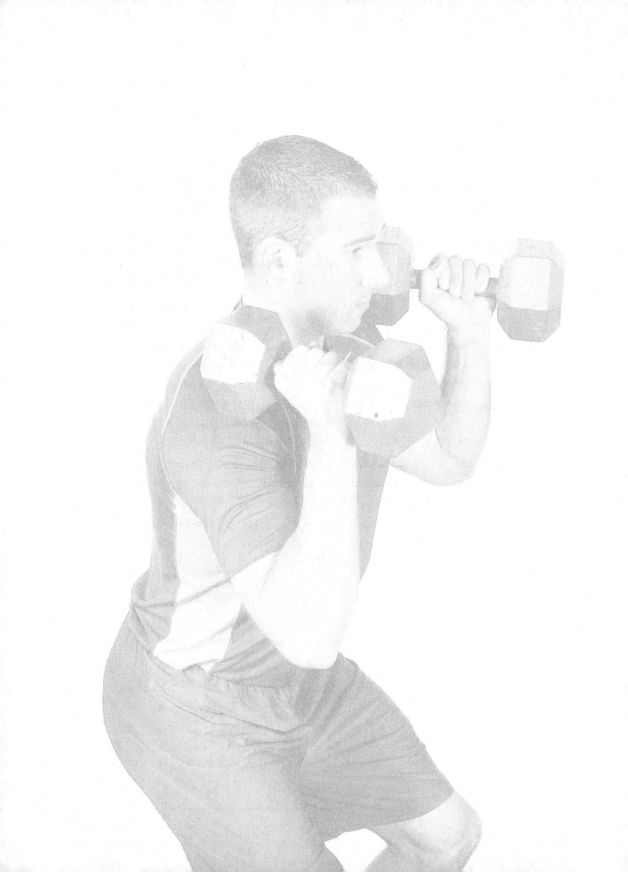

CHAPTER 1

WHY STRONGER IS BETTER

Go to any local gym, make your way into the free weights room, and you'll see the same thing. The majority of the men there are performing familiar exercises, including the flat bench press, the EZ-bar biceps curl, and the cable triceps pushdown. If you count the number of times each of these movements is repeated before a rest is taken, the final tally will be 10, give or take a rep or two, more often than not. Finally, you may also notice that each of the exercisers in the room is concentrating on one or two areas of his body—doing exercises for his chest and shoulders, perhaps, or just his arms. (Those concentrating on their legs will surely be in the minority.)

All of these behaviors that you will observe in the gym—any gym—are classic features of the bodybuilding approach to resistance training, of which the purpose is to maximize muscle growth. This approach is almost ubiquitous among men who lift weights in gyms. Yet there are, and have been throughout history, other types of resistance exercise that serve other purposes. The modern sport of Olympic weightlifting involves high-speed overhead barbell lifts that are based on the feats of strength performed by the Olympians of ancient Greece (which they did with forms of resistance other than barbells, of course). Soldiers have performed calisthenics exercises—body-weight resistance movements—to enhance functional strength and muscular endurance for centuries. And in my sport, powerlifting, the competitive lifts (bench press, deadlift, squat) are familiar enough, but the way we train them (very heavy loads and low reps) is not, nor are many of the supporting exercises we do in training.

Why does the bodybuilding approach so dominate recreational resistance training, even though it is not the ideal approach for the recreational weightlifter? The answer is simple: because bodybuilders, beginning with Charles Atlas in the 1920s and peaking with Arnold Schwarzenegger in the 1970s and 1980s, were the ones who made recreational weightlifting popular.

The problem with this type of training is that it's inefficient and is really designed for men who are capable of achieving an absurd level of muscle size that most men cannot achieve and probably wouldn't want even if they could attain it. Also, traditional bodybuilding methods are derivatives of programs from lifters who were big-time steroid users, so they seldom work for the average guy. Given a choice, most men would rather be the strongest man in town than the largest, but the bodybuilding mentality has been so dominant for so long that, until now, nobody has given guys the choice.

Not only is strength a better goal than size for most men, but training for maximum strength is a much better way than training for muscle size alone to get all of the results men seek from weightlifting. Training for maximum strength has several advantages over bodybuilding-style training. Specifically, maximum strength training is:

1. MORE TIME-EFFICIENT

Bodybuilding-style training is a high-volume (i.e., time-consuming) approach to resistance training. In that approach, individual muscle groups are isolated and trained individually. Consequently, large numbers of exercises are required to cover the whole body. By contrast, maximum strength training emphasizes "compound movements" that challenge multiple muscle groups, so the participant can cover his whole body with fewer exercises. In addition, maximum strength involves heavier loads, so the muscles reach an appropriate level of fatigue more quickly (with fewer sets and repetitions). With today's busy schedules, every second is precious. If you're like most guys, you want to get maximum results in minimum time spent in the gym. Maximum strength training is the ideal resistance training method for the time-crunched.

Many professional bodybuilders spend two to three hours a day in the gym, including a morning session and an afternoon session, six days a week. I'm guessing that those of you who don't lift weights for a living don't have that kind of time to devote. Fortunately, you can realize 100 percent of your genetic potential for strength by going to the gym just four times a week for approximately an hour per session. And that's exactly what you will do on the Maximum Strength Program. Heck, I compete as a high-level powerlifter and I don't train much more than that.

2. MORE USEFUL IN THE REAL WORLD

In recent years there has been a sea change in the world of fitness that is often referred to as the *functional fitness revolution*. Personal trainers have switched their focus from designing and prescribing workout programs that are intended primarily to improve appearance to designing and prescribing programs that are intended primarily to improve the body's performance in life. Most types of exercise improve both appearance and function, but some types improve function more than others. Training for maximum strength improves function and performance much more effectively than bodybuilding-style training.

Pound for pound, powerlifters, who train for strength, are usually stronger than bodybuilders, who train for size. Maximum strength exercises not only involve heavier loads than bodybuilding exercises, and thus boost strength more, but also require more balance and coordination. As a result, the fitness gains made in the gym through maximum strength training have greater functional carryover to real-life activities such as moving furniture and pushing stalled cars.

In addition, if you participate in any type of sport, maximum strength is a far superior method of conditioning than bodybuilding to improve your sports performance. Almost every sport requires power, or the ability to express strength quickly. For example, any sport that involves running requires power, because power is the basis of sprint speed. Bodybuilding entails slow lifts that do not increase power. But the Maximum Strength Program includes a number of high-speed lifts that will produce dramatic increases in your muscle power as well as your maximum strength.

A basic test of power we'll use is the broad jump. The more force you can apply to the ground with your feet, and the more quickly you can generate this force, the farther you can broad-jump. That's why I've included the broad jump among the Moving Day strength (and power) tests you will perform at the end of the Maximum Strength Program (and among the pretests you'll do before you start the program). This test will enable you to measure your power gains. But you'll also feel them on the basketball court, on the mountain bike trails, or wherever else you might benefit from having a little extra power.

3. MORE MOTIVATING

Imagine you have a bad case of hemorrhoids. (Bear with me; there's a point to this analogy.) Every time you sit down, it's like impaling yourself on a hot poker. Your primary-care physician checked them out and said they're going to have to be surgically lanced. You have a choice of two doctors to perform the procedure. The first doctor studied hemorrhoids for two years in school. The second doctor studied for only one year but also passed a stringent test of hemorrhoid-lancing ability. Which doctor would you choose?

Personally, I would entrust my aching tuchus to the test passer, not only because I have proof that he knows how to do the job, but also because I know human psychology well enough to know he probably learned twice as much in his one year of study as the other guy learned in two. When there are tests to pass and deadlines to meet, we tend to work harder and more effectively. When there are no tests to pass or deadlines to meet, we slack off, even if we don't think we're slacking off.

What do hypothetical hemorrhoid surgeons have to do with your muscles? I'll tell you. There's a huge difference between "working out" and "training." When the results you seek from exercise are not clearly defined, then you're merely *working out*. Your program lacks direction, focus, and progression. Consequently, although you may put a lot of time and energy into your sessions, your progress is minimal, and at times it might even be hard to tell whether you're making progress or not.

However, when you take specific performance goals to the gym, you are *training*. Chasing concrete and measurable goals has a way of making one's program more focused, more progressive, and ultimately more effective. When I was lifting weights only to look better, I was merely working out. I was like that hemorrhoid surgeon with twice the schooling but half the ability, because he had never had to buckle down for a test. But when I became a powerlifter, I started training. I became like the test-passing hemorrhoid surgeon, busting his ass (so to speak) for a date with destiny.

For most guys, the all-too-common goal of "getting bigger" is too fuzzy to motivate actions that will result in any real progress. Countless lifters have "bulked up" only to find that they've added too much body fat, and then decide to "get cut." Once they've lost some body fat, they realize that they're right back where they started; there's been no significant change in spite of all that hard work. It's like driving around the world just to move your parking spot from the north side of the street to the south side.

By contrast, a performance goal such as "I want to increase my maximum strength in four specific lifts in 16 weeks" incorporates the specificity and measurability that are needed to make significant advancement. Success and progress are objectively defined, there's a specific endpoint, and the whole project has the purposeful structure of a contest. What do you do after you have achieved this performance goal? Set another one!

Competitive athletes are the role models for training instead of working out, because measurable, time-bound performance goals are built into every sport. Nonathletes who wish to achieve a better body need to take a page from competitive athletes' book by setting performance goals and training specifically to achieve them. It's the best way to make real progress; subjective goals such as "looking better" just don't cut it.

I broke free from the go-nowhere cycle of working out to get bigger by becoming a competitive powerlifter. If you're caught in the same cycle, you don't necessarily have to sign up for a powerlifting meet, but you should follow the example of competitive lifters like me and borrow the strength sports' built-in performance goal: increasing the amount of weight you can lift.

4. A FASTER WAY TO BUILD MUSCLE MASS (POTENTIALLY)

At the elite level, bodybuilders, who train specifically for muscle growth, almost always have larger muscles than powerlifters, who train specifically for muscle strength. But for the average gym member, training for maximum strength can actually result in faster gains in muscle mass than bodybuilding-style training. You see, many successful bodybuilders start with a solid strength foundation, something very few everyday gym goers possess. Additionally, getting the full muscle-boosting effect of bodybuilding-style training requires a level of time commitment that is impossible for the average gym member. On a manageable schedule of four one-hour sessions per week, maximum strength training will almost certainly produce greater mass gains than bodybuilding-style training.

Even if your ultimate goal is to maximize your muscle mass, completing the Maximum Strength Program will move you closer to that goal than continuing to train in the same way you've been training. I train a number of bodybuilders, and I put each of them through a strength-focused phase of training that is similar to the Maximum Strength Program, and the end result is always the same: Their muscles get bigger.

The reason is that lack of strength often becomes the limiting factor for muscle growth in bodybuilders. Very generally speaking, bodybuilders increase their muscle size by increasing the amount of weight they can lift 6–10 times (that is, by increasing their 6–10-rep maxes, or 6–10RM) in various movements. However, if *all* of your training involves sets of 6–10 repetitions, more or less, as is the case for many bodybuilders, before long you will hit a plateau. Without any fresh stimulus for further gains, your 6–10-rep maxes will stop increasing, and so will your muscle size.

The surest way to bust through this plateau is to do some maximum strength training that increases your 1-rep max (1RM) in various lifts. Increasing your 1RM will automatically increase your 6–10RM more-or-less proportionally. In addition, your added maximal strength will give you a foundation to increase your 6–10RM even further when you return to emphasizing higher-rep training.

5. BETTER FOR YOUR HEALTH AND LONGEVITY

New research has demonstrated that muscle strength declines significantly with age, and that increasing one's muscle strength is one of the most effective ways to slow the overall aging process. Sarcopenia, or the aging-related decline in muscle mass, is known to greatly reduce performance in daily living activities in the elderly and is also linked to obesity, diabetes, heart disease, osteoporosis, and Alzheimer's disease. Muscle mass typically begins to decline after age 30, while muscle strength typically starts a downward spiral at approximately age 50.

Any type of consistent resistance training will slow sarcopenia, enhance functional performance in one's golden years, and reduce degenerative disease risk—but maximum strength training will do all of these things better than bodybuilding-style training. A recent study from the University of Pittsburgh found that greater muscle *strength* was strongly correlated with lower mortality risk in a population of elderly men and women, while greater muscle *size* was not.

Interestingly, recent research has shown that the functional decline in activities of daily living that is seen in older persons has more to do with loss of muscle power (or the capacity to generate force quickly) than with loss of either muscle mass or muscle strength. The classic example of the need for muscle power in daily life is making rapid bodily adjustments to avoid falling after tripping. Those who maintain muscle power in their golden years are less likely to trip in the first place and less likely to fall when they do trip than their peers who lose muscle power, even if they retain strength and mass. They will also have an easier time getting up and down stairs, climbing into and out of cars, doing yardwork, and participating in any vigorous recreational activities, such as kinky sex. As I mentioned above, maximum strength training is a much better power builder than bodybuilding-style resistance training.

6. A BETTER WAY TO BUILD SELF-CONFIDENCE

Those who actively seek maximum muscle growth in the gym are sometimes motivated by insecurity and lack of self-confidence. The famous Charles Atlas comic book advertisements that started the bodybuilding craze were so effective precisely because they preyed upon the insecurities of boys and young men—fears of being unattractive to females and easily bullied by other males.

Unfortunately, achieving muscle growth doesn't always improve one's self-confidence, because it is all about appearance instead of substance. A man who needs to look intimidating to feel confident is not really confident. He's like the dog that barks loudly because he knows his bite is weak.

Maximum strength training is a better way to build genuine self-confidence because it gives men real substance for confidence and encourages them to stop caring about having an intimidating appearance. The most self-assured man in a crowded room is not the man who looks the toughest; he's the man who actually *is* the toughest. Psychologists have discovered that the bedrock of confidence is something called self-efficacy, or taking pride in what one is able to do. Being able to lift heavy objects is a fundamental ability in which any man can take pride. Increasing your ability to lift heavy objects is therefore a sure way to increase your sense of self-efficacy and confidence. It may seem like a small thing, but shifting your mind-set away from the appearance orientation of getting huge to the substance orientation of getting strong could give your emotional well-being a big boost.

A STRONG CASE FOR STRENGTH

In summary, maximum strength training is more time-efficient, more useful in the real world, more motivating, better for your health and longevity, a more effective means of building muscles mass, and a better confidence-builder than traditional bodybuilding methods. While we still borrow many great strategies from bodybuilding, most weekend warriors would be wise to make the switch from bodybuilding-style training to maximum strength training.

But what exactly is the difference between muscle size and muscle strength, and why do the training methods used in the Maximum Strength Program increase strength more effectively than other methods? The next chapter will answer these questions.

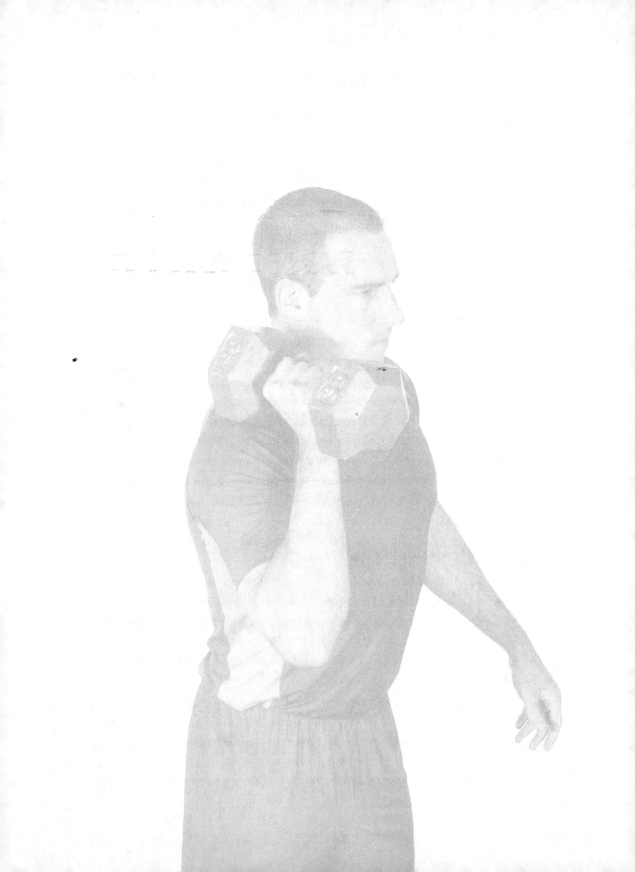

CHAPTER 2

BUILDING STRENGTH

One of my distance-consulting clients is an up-and-coming British golfer named David Hills. Besides being a gifted athlete, Dave is also an avid student of the art and science of sports training and conditioning. Recently, Dave trekked across the Atlantic to train in person with me for a few weeks at my facility in Boston. While he was here, he made a point of coming by to observe a training session that I did with three athletes I was helping to prepare for upcoming professional football combines.

Among these players was a linebacker who stood 6 feet tall and weighed 237 pounds. I myself am only 5 feet 8 inches tall, and I tipped the scale at 185 pounds at the time. Standing next to that gridiron goliath, I probably looked like a child. So Dave was utterly amazed to see me out-bench-press the linebacker by 55 pounds.

"That's amazing," he said.

"Not really, if you think about it," I replied. "You're just seeing the difference between size and strength."

David Hills is not alone in casually assuming that muscle size and muscle strength are more or less the same thing. Of course, everyone knows that smaller guys are sometimes stronger than bigger guys. But by and large, we expect larger muscles to exhibit greater strength. And more importantly, we expect that in any given individual, muscle size and muscle strength will always increase in equal proportion. But this is not the case.

Suppose you know two guys, Chad and Brad, who happen to be identical twins. One day they tell you they've decided to go away to separate 16-week conditioning camps, where they will undergo two different types of training. At the time of their departure, their bodies are indistinguishable. But when they come back 16 weeks later, the two brothers look quite different. Chad has put on a substantial amount of muscle—at least 10 pounds of it. His arms, chest, and legs look puffy and pumped. Brad has also put on some muscle, but not as much—perhaps 6 pounds. Yet his muscles have a much denser and harder look than Chad's.

Now, which of these two twins would you wager increased his maximum deadlift, squat, and bench press more during the preceding 16 weeks? Most people would guess Chad—but I wouldn't bet against Brad. By the time you finish reading this chapter, you'll know why.

THE DEFINITION OF STRENGTH

In a famous U.S. Supreme Court decision, Justice Potter Stewart argued that he could not define pornography; however, he wrote, "I know it when I see it." I'm sure you do, your honor.

The concept of strength is also hard to define, but for a different reason: because there are many forms of strength, each specific to a particular function. For our purposes, we can define human physical strength simply as the capacity to move a load against resistance. The load can be one's own body, a shovel full of snow, a weighted barbell, or many other things. The resistance is usually the force of gravity, which is inseparable from the load, because the weight of a load is defined as the amount of force that is required to move that load away from the center of the earth. But there are also other, gravity-independent forms of resistance, such as the elastic resistance that must be overcome to stretch a resistance band and the frictional resistance that must be overcome to push a tackling sled.

Many factors contribute to human physical strength, and not all of them have to do with muscles. For example, having short limbs makes certain strength tasks easier to perform by reducing the distance a load has to travel. I have long arms and legs for my height, which put me at a disadvantage when I bench-press and squat (but help when I deadlift).

The two major muscular properties that affect strength are the muscle's cross-sectional area and neuromuscular efficiency. Muscle cross-sectional area refers to the thickness of a muscle. As a general rule, the thicker a given muscle becomes, the more forcefully it can contract. This is the case, in part, because thicker muscles have thicker muscle fibers, and thicker muscle fibers usually contain a larger number of contractile proteins, which are the fundamental mechanisms of muscle contraction. Adding contractile proteins to your muscle fibers is sort of like adding pullers to your side of the rope in a tug-of-war.

Neuromuscular efficiency is a broad concept that refers to the contribution of brain-muscle communications to strength performance. Every muscle contraction starts in the brain. A part of your brain called the motor center sends an electrical signal through your spine and motor nerves into your muscle fibers, causing them to shorten. Training produces changes in this system that enable you to contract your muscles faster, more forcefully, and more efficiently. If you think of the brain's role in muscle contractions as being like that of a drill sergeant commanding a platoon of muscle fibers to contract, then this increase in neural drive is like turning up the volume of the command from a whisper to a shout.

Gains in neuromuscular efficiency happen independently of muscle growth. That's why you can't always predict how strong someone is from the size of his muscles. A person with relatively small muscles and a high level of neuromuscular efficiency often can outlift a person with larger muscles and a lower level of neuromuscular efficiency.

The ideal type of training to increase a muscle's cross-sectional area is different from the ideal type of training to increase neuromuscular efficiency. When you're a beginner, pretty much any kind of training will increase both your muscle size and your neuromuscular efficiency. As you increase the volume of weightlifting you do or the amount of weight you lift, or both, you will continue to increase the cross-sectional area of your muscles and your neuromuscular efficiency. However, as you become more experienced, you come to a point where it simply isn't possible to train to maximize both the size and the strength of your muscles simultaneously. The reason is that you cannot truly maximize the volume of weightlifting you do and the amount of weight you lift simultaneously. If

(handwritten annotation: → Aka Muscle Size)

(handwritten annotation: → Aka Muscle Strength)

you want to maximize your training volume, you have to limit the amount of weight you lift, so your muscles don't become exhausted too quickly. But if you want to maximize the amount of weight you lift, you have to limit your training volume, because lifting very heavy weights will fatigue your muscles faster.

For reasons that I will explain below, doing a high volume of weightlifting with moderately heavy weights is the most effective way to increase muscles' cross-sectional area. Lifting very heavy weights is the best way to increase neuromuscular efficiency. So if you choose to emphasize volume over weight in your training, you will eventually reach a point where the volume of training you do for size gains actually comes at the expense of neuromuscular efficiency, causing your strength to plateau. Therefore, if your goal is to increase your maximal strength as much as possible, you need to train in a way that balances muscle growth with gains in neuromuscular efficiency—and that's where I come in!

WHAT MAKES MUSCLES GROW?

Scientists are still trying to figure out the mechanisms of muscle growth, that is, precisely how hormones, genes, immune cells, and other factors cooperate in response to training to increase the size of existing muscle fibers and to cause new muscle fibers to develop. We've learned a lot within the past few years, but many aspects of the process are still shrouded in mystery. What we know much more about is the types of training that promote muscle growth most effectively. Fortunately for those who are seeking maximal muscle growth, it is possible to know what works without having the foggiest notion of why the hell it works!

The two training factors that have the greatest impact on muscle growth are load and sets/reps. To put it in terms any kindergartner can understand: If you want big muscles, you have to lift heavy weights and you have to lift them many times. This training approach is known as the *repetition method*. Lifting heavy loads is required to stimulate muscle growth because heavy loads cause far more muscle tissue disruption than lighter loads, and muscle tissue disruption is a key initiator of the adaptive processes that make muscles grow. Of course, lifting a heavy weight six times will cause more tissue disruption than lifting it three times, and completing two sets of six heavy lifts will cause more tissue disruption than completing one set—and that's why volume is important for muscle growth, as well.

The catch is that load and reps are inversely related. The more weight you lift, the fewer times you can lift it. Likewise, the more times you plan to lift a weight, the lighter that weight must be. You can work around this issue in various ways: by performing multiple sets with rest breaks between them, by pairing relatively unrelated exercises to avoid overlap, and by training frequently—but the fact remains that you can achieve only so much volume without sacrificing the load.

Now, by definition, you can lift your one-repetition maximum (1RM) load for any given movement only one time. Sure, you might be able to lift it again after a few minutes of rest, but at most you can complete only a handful of 1RM lifts separated by full recoveries before you're exhausted. The cause of exhaustion in such cases is nervous system fatigue, which essentially means your brain, spinal cord, and peripheral nerves refuse to "tell" your muscles to continue working at maximum capacity. When you lift maximal loads, nervous system fatigue sets in before muscle tissue disruption reaches the levels it reaches when you lift somewhat lighter loads more times. This is one reason why you have to find a middle ground between load and volume if you want to maximize muscle growth.

Muscles contain two basic types of muscle fibers: type I fibers, which are endurance specialists, and type II fibers, which are strength specialists. Bodybuilding-type training presents the muscles with a greater endurance challenge than maximum strength training does, because bodybuilding-type training involves lifting lighter weights more times. In other words, bodybuilding-type training challenges the type I muscle fibers a little more than maximum strength training does, while maximum strength training challenges the type II fibers more. Interestingly, research has shown that bodybuilding-type training causes the type I muscle fibers to grow more than maximum strength training does. This may be another reason bodybuilders have found that high-volume training with moderately heavy loads is most effective for muscle growth.

Bodybuilders certainly are not endurance athletes in the sense that distance runners and cyclists are. However, the primary reason bodybuilders tend to have larger muscles than powerlifters and Olympic weightlifters is that bodybuilding-type training stimulates structural adaptations in the muscles that increase both strength and short-term endurance, whereas maximal strength training tends to increase strength alone. The only structural adaptation that's really needed to increase maximal strength is an increase in the number and concentration of contractile proteins in the muscles. However, to increase their endurance—even relatively short-term, anaerobic endurance—the muscles also need to store more fuel, acid buffers, fluid, and other things that help them resist fatigue. And this is exactly what we see when we look inside the muscles of bodybuilders. For example, studies have shown that bodybuilding-type training increases the amount of muscle glycogen (the primary fuel for sustained high-intensity exercise) stored in the muscles almost as much as marathon training does. Since the muscles store nearly three grams of water for every gram of glycogen they store, this adaptation tends to increase the size of muscle cells.

When we look inside the muscles of powerlifters and Olympic weightlifters (especially lightweight competitors), we see a greater concentration of contractile proteins than we do in bodybuilders, but smaller amounts of all the other "junk" that increases endurance and cell volume. Since contractile proteins are much denser than the other junk, the muscles of strength athletes take on a dense look, while those of bodybuilders look puffier. The fact that the contractile proteins are more closely connected to maximal strength than the other junk explains why I wouldn't hesitate to put my money on a denser Brad to bench-press, deadlift, and squat more than his bigger twin brother, Chad.

due to glycogen, water, etc.

Maximal strength training has its place in the training programs of bodybuilders and others seeking maximum muscle growth. For that matter, corrective strength training, high-repetition low-load "foundation" training, and other types of training also have their place in such programs. You can't take any type of fitness very far—be it muscle size, maximal strength, speed, endurance, or anything else—without variation in your training methods. Clearly, though, the specific type of training that is most effective for increasing muscle size is, again, high volume with moderately heavy loads (e.g., multiple sets of 6 to 12 repetitions with 6 to 12RM loads). Other standard bodybuilding methods that serve to maximize the training volume with such loads include selecting exercises that attempt to "isolate" individual muscle groups, performing multiple exercises for a given muscle group within a workout, training only a few muscle groups per training session, and training each muscle group frequently.

WHAT MAKES MUSCLES STRONG?

As I mentioned above, two factors contribute to gains in muscle strength: increasing muscle cross-sectional area (that is, increasing muscle size) and improved neuromuscular efficiency. The most important factor in muscle strength gains is improved neuromuscular efficiency. Beginning weightlifters always become stronger before their muscles become measurably larger because of improvements in neuromuscular efficiency. Specifically, the brain quickly learns to send stronger contraction signals to the muscles in response to the challenges imposed by strength protocols.

There is evidence that, beyond the beginner level, further improvements in neuromuscular efficiency are largely responsible for further strength gains, all the way to the point where an individual reaches his genetic limit for strength. There are three specific adaptations to training that enhance neuromuscular efficiency:

1. **MORE MUSCLE INVOLVEMENT:** When you contract a muscle, you might assume that all of the tissue in that muscle is actively involved in the contraction. But it's not. In fact, the average beginning weightlifter is able to activate only half the tissue in a given muscle when contracting it with maximum force. Training quickly increases the amount of muscle tissue your brain can activate.

2. **FASTER MUSCLE ACTIVATION:** Training also increases the speed at which electrical signals travel from the brain's motor center to the muscles, enabling the muscles to contract more powerfully.

3. **BETTER COORDINATION:** The brain learns to use "co-contraction"—or the activation of muscles other than the prime movers in a given lift—to stabilize joints better and improve the efficiency of joint movements. It also learns to relax antagonist muscles that inhibit force production in the desired direction of movement.

While beginners can improve their strength using virtually any type of resistance training involving loads greater than 40 percent of 1RM, continued strength gains require further increases in training load to 70 percent of 1RM and above (all the way to 90 to 100 percent in more advanced lifters). In other words, to truly maximize your muscle strength, you must *use* your maximal muscle strength in training. Only maximal-effort lifts are capable of stimulating the primarily neural adaptations that serve to increase maximal strength beyond a certain point. This approach to developing muscle tension to increase maximal strength is known as—drum roll, please—the *maximal effort method.*

In addition to the repetition and maximal effort methods, there is a third and rather different training method of developing muscle tension that is also effective in increasing maximal strength. It's called the *dynamic effort method.* Unlike the maximal effort method, which entails lifting heavy loads of 85 to 100 percent of 1RM, the dynamic effort method entails lifting lighter loads, typically ranging between 35 and 75 percent of 1RM, at a rapid speed. How does the dynamic effort method contribute to building maximal strength? The answer has to do with time—and speed.

In order to lift the maximum load you are capable of lifting in any given movement, you must attempt to lift (or more precisely, accelerate) the load as quickly as possible; this phenomenon is known as *compensatory acceleration.* The reason is that a neural command from the brain's motor centers telling the muscles to contract (shorten) as fast as possible is required to activate the largest number of muscle fibers simultaneously, and this rapid activation is in turn required to produce maximal force. However, there is a difference between the *intent* to lift a load quickly—which is essential for maximal strength performance—and the ability to actually contract the muscles quickly based on that intent. It all depends on the size of the load you're attempting to lift and the specific nature of the strength task you're performing.

Consider the example of a vertical jump versus a heavy barbell squat. In both movements, maximum performance requires the intent to exert as much force from the feet into the ground as quickly as possible. In the case of the vertical jump, because the load is mere body weight, the muscles can, in fact, contract very quickly, allowing force to be sent into the ground very quickly and returned just as fast, sending the athlete skyward. But in the case of the heavy squat, the large load prevents the muscles from contracting quickly, even though they are trying to contract just as fast as in the vertical jump.

Research has shown that somewhat different neural and muscular adaptations result from dynamic effort training than from maximal effort training. (By the way, you can perform almost any lift as a dynamic effort lift by selecting an appropriate load and cranking up the speed of movement. For example, the barbell squat becomes a dynamic effort lift when a 50 percent of 1RM load is lifted two to four times at a rapid tempo.) If you want to optimize your performance in strength tests that allow fast muscle contractions, it is essential that you incorporate dynamic effort training into your program. The set of strength tests with which the Maximum Strength Program culminates on Moving Day includes one such test: a broad jump, making dynamic effort training a requirement within the program. Still, dynamic effort training can also contribute to performance in other strength tests, such as the maximal squat, as long as it is combined with maximal effort training in a complementary way. For this reason, the dynamic effort component of the Maximum Strength Program is not limited to exercises that are specifically designed to enhance broad-jump performance.

In addition to its greater emphasis on the maximal effort method and the dynamic effort method versus the repetition method, training for maximal strength also differs from bodybuilding-type training in its greater emphasis on whole-body movements. Most of the traditional tests of strength are whole-body exercises. Naturally, in order to increase your performance in such tests as much as possible, you need to emphasize whole-body movements over isolation movements in training. For example, machine hamstring curls will do very little to improve your deadlift performance, even though the hamstrings act as prime movers in the deadlift, because unlike machine hamstring curls, the deadlift requires the hamstrings to work in coordination with many other muscle groups.

This is not to say that isolation movements cannot serve a purpose in maximal strength training. Just as there is a place for maximal strength lifts in bodybuilding-type training, there is also a place for isolation movements here and there in maximal strength training. Specifically, certain isolation movements are beneficial in correcting muscle imbalances and strengthening stabilizing muscles to create a sound frame that can better handle the heavy loads and whole-body movements emphasized later in the training process.

Fatigue occurs faster in sessions emphasizing whole-body movements than it does in workouts emphasizing isolation movements for various muscle groups. This is the second reason powerlifters and Olympic weightlifters, who emphasize whole-body movements, typically don't spend as much time in the gym as bodybuilders, who emphasize isolation exercises. The first reason, you will recall, is that training with very heavy loads causes nervous system fatigue fairly quickly. (To be perfectly accurate, many Olympic weightlifters and powerlifters actually perform longer training sessions than bodybuilders, but more of that training time is necessarily spent resting between lifts and performing ancillary training, such as dynamic flexibility work.)

THE RECIPE FOR STRENGTH

Taking into account these two important fatigue factors, the Maximum Strength Program entails only 4 (ball-busting) resistance-training sessions per week—far fewer than the 6 to 12 weekly resistance workouts that serious bodybuilders do. The loads are mostly heavier than those used in bodybuilding workouts, and there is also more dynamic effort work and a greater emphasis on whole-body movements than in the typical bodybuilding program. These features make the Maximum Strength Program ideally suited to increase your maximal strength—which, as you now understand, is rather different from maximum muscle size—as much as possible in 16 weeks. That said, let me reiterate that the methods on which the Maximum Strength Program is based still build appreciable muscle mass, just like the bodybuilding-type training you're probably used to, which means you will very likely gain some muscle mass on the program to go along with the excellent performance gains you experience. The next chapter provides a detailed overview of the program.

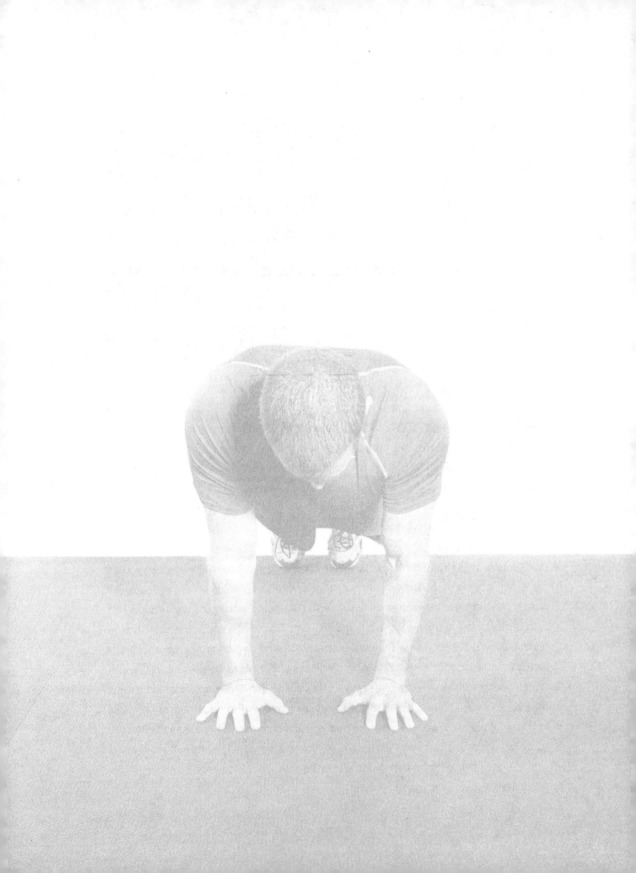

CHAPTER 3

MAXIMUM STRENGTH PROGRAM OVERVIEW

The Maximum Strength Program, which you're about to start, is loosely modeled on a powerlifting training cycle. It is 16 weeks long and culminates in a set of four maximal performance lifts plus a maximal power test (broad jump) on the final day—your own private Powerlifting World Championship. Your goals are to lift as much weight as possible in each of these four lifts and to jump as far as possible in the power test. The training that you do throughout the program will develop your strength step by step from where you are now to where you want to be. This training is very different from—and more effective than— the type of training you would do if your only goal were to "get bigger." What's more, because the training is focused on a meaningful, measurable goal and enables continual progress-monitoring along the way, it encourages a competitive, performance-oriented mind-set that enhances motivation and training enjoyment and makes it easy to work hard, guaranteeing you even better results.

MOVING DAY

Powerlifters and other competitive athletes work backward. They start by setting the goal of achieving maximum performance in some future competition. Once this destination is chosen, it's relatively straightforward to create a map and plan a route between Point A (the athlete's current fitness level) and Point B (peak performance in competition).

The same is true of the Maximum Strength Program. The name I've given to the five-movement self-competition that marks the program's destination is Moving Day. This name has a special meaning. At no other time in everyday life is great strength more useful than when you're moving your furniture and other worldly possessions from one home to another. Thus, the name Moving Day calls attention to the real-world benefits that the program offers. The unofficial motto of the Maximum Strength Program is this: "Kick ass on Moving Day!"

The four maximal lifts you'll do on Moving Day are the box squat, bench press, deadlift, and three-repetition chin-up. The box squat is a modified version of the standard barbell squat that's used in powerlifting. We'll detail proper execution later, but the basic idea is to use the box to deload in the bottom position, teach you to "sit back" into your squats, and verify that you've hit proper depth on the squat (thighs parallel to the floor). The bench press and deadlift you'll do on Moving Day are the same as those done in powerlifting competitions. The three-repetition chin-up test is a nontraditional strength test, but I like it because, unlike the other lifts, it's a test of relative strength, or strength-to-weight ratio, in which the lightweights can get their revenge on those 500-pounders who squat Buicks because they bounce their massive bellies off their thighs in the bottom position! You simply perform three chin-ups while carrying the maximum external weight (in the form of weight plates attached to a weight belt) that you can carry.

Moving Day also features a "bonus" power test: a standing broad jump. It used to be an Olympic event, believe it or not. It was actually done in the buff—which you are welcome to do, too—but only at home, with the shades pulled down. Either way, the broad jump is a great relative-power test for the lower body and an accurate predictor of athletic ability.

But wait: How will you know that your performance in these lifts actually improved during the 16-week Maximum Strength Program? Simple. Before you begin the program, you'll check them with a pretest: Packing Day!

The training program will prepare you fairly specifically for maximum improvement in these lifts, but not quite as specifically as I would have you train if there were fame and prize money at stake. The real objective of the training is to increase your general strength—as well as your overall fitness and health—as much as possible in 16 weeks. Therefore you'll do plenty of single-leg training, core stability work, rotational drills, overhead pressing, scapular stability training, dynamic flexibility, and even some energy workouts (a modified version of what the unwashed masses call cardio).

PROGRAM STRUCTURE

The 16-week duration of the Maximum Strength Program is not accidental. On the one hand, 16 weeks is a long enough time period to make substantial strength gains. On the other hand, it's short enough to keep your motivation level high. As powerful as they are, performance goals lose some of their motivating force if their time horizon is too far in the distance. The way to keep your motivation level high over the long term is to set a new short-term performance goal after you achieve a goal. In Chapter 12 I will share some tips for keeping your momentum going beyond Moving Day.

The weekly training schedule includes four strength sessions per week, plus two or three optional energy (i.e., cardio) workouts. Two of the four weekly strength sessions focus predominantly on the upper body, and the other two primarily address the lower body. The weekly schedule is as follows:

MONDAY: Strength (lower body)
TUESDAY: Energy (optional)
WEDNESDAY: Strength (upper body)
THURSDAY: Energy (optional)
FRIDAY: Strength (lower body)
SATURDAY: Strength (upper body)
SUNDAY: Rest (or energy)

While I know of many people who have had success with programs that have them lifting anywhere from two to six days per week, I've found that the above schedule works best for the majority of lifters. Training less frequently has proven beneficial to some, but training more frequently is rarely more effective, as it takes the central nervous system (CNS) a few days to recover from very-high-intensity strength work—even if the muscles are feeling "good to go." It's very important that your CNS recover enough between training sessions so that you are able to perform at a high enough level in the next session to achieve the requisite loading—and so that you avoid accumulating excessive, chronic fatigue.

ENERGY WORKOUTS

Energy work is tricky for those who are training to increase maximum strength. Sustained aerobic exercise stimulates muscular adaptations that conflict with the neural and muscular adaptations that are required to increase maximum strength. This "interference phenomenon" is well documented in the scientific literature. For example, in a study from the University of Alberta, Canada, 40 volunteers engaged in 12 weeks of either strength training alone, cardio training alone, or a combination of both. Subjects on the pure strength-training program gained significantly more strength and muscle mass than those on the combined program, even though the hybrid training subjects did just as much lifting.

Interestingly, the pure-strength subjects in this study experienced a threefold greater increase in the size of their type I muscle fibers than the hybrid trainers. These muscle fibers are most responsive to cardio training, which causes them to increase their oxygen-using capacity. They can also respond to strength training with increases in size and strength. But if too much cardio training is combined with strength training, the slow-twitch fibers will adapt in the direction of their endurance specialty rather than in the direction of strength, which seems to be what happened to the hybrid trainers in the study.

Many powerlifters, fearing the interference phenomenon, avoid all cardio training. I don't think that's necessary. A sensible approach to cardio training will actually complement your strength training nicely. For example, one research group found that when the intensity of cardiovascular exercise was kept below 70 percent of heart-rate reserve, strength gains were not impaired in a combined aerobic and resistance-training group compared to a resistance-training-only group. Perhaps more convincing is the fact that some of the most successful powerlifters and strongman athletes in the world incorporate cardio sessions into their training with no apparent ill effects. A properly planned and executed cardio session may enhance recovery from recent strength training via increased blood flow. Also, nontraditional cardio approaches, such as low-intensity resistance training, may complement strength training by increasing neuromuscular coordination in relevant movement patterns.

In addition, energy work offers major health benefits. It reduces body fat stores, enhances brain health, reduces arterial plaque formation, increases insulin sensitivity, and boosts longevity.

The most appropriate way to incorporate cardio training into the Maximum Strength Program depends on your body type—or, more exactly, your somatotype. I will provide specific somatotype-based energy workout guidelines in Chapters 6 through 9. Generally speaking, endomorphs—or those who tend to add fat mass easily and struggle to put on lean muscle mass—need to include more cardio work to optimize their body composition and relative strength. If you're an endomorph, I recommend that you perform three or four cardio sessions per week throughout the program. These might include some appropriately scheduled high-intensity interval training (HIIT) sessions, some low-intensity cardiovascular work (at 60 to 70 percent of maximum heart rate), and/or some low-intensity, higher-rep resistance-training circuits on non-strength-training days. The latter two modalities offer the additional benefit of facilitating recovery from the higher-intensity exercise that characterizes the Maximum Strength Program.

Mesomorphs, however, are lucky enough to gain muscle relatively easily and are generally able to keep body fat in check with only a few (one to three) cardio sessions per week. Generally speaking, if these guys are interested in really enhancing maximal strength, they should avoid HIIT and go with only the low-intensity cardio and the low-intensity, higher-rep resistance-training circuits, both of which promote blood flow and enhance recovery.

Ectomorphs are naturally skinny individuals who struggle to gain muscle mass because of their lightning-fast metabolism. This class of individuals doesn't need much cardio at all—two sessions per week at most—and it should mostly come from low-intensity, higher-rep resistance-training circuits.

As you can see, I want you to avoid that 70 to 90 percent of max heart rate range at all costs; that's where strength gains are inhibited! Following are brief descriptions of the three types of cardio approaches I'm including in the Maximum Strength Program (depending on somatotype).

High-Intensity Interval Training (HIIT)

Choose any cardio-training modality: running, swimming, rowing, cycling, elliptical training, and so on. Warm up with five minutes at a low intensity, and then increase your effort to maximum (relative to the interval duration) for 10 to 30 seconds. Depending on your choice of activity, you can increase the effort level not only by increasing your pace but also by increasing the resistance level. For example, if you're riding a bike, you may switch to a high gear ratio (outdoors) or a high resistance level (stationary bike). After completing a high-intensity interval, slow back down to your warm-up pace for 30 to 120 seconds for "active recovery." Complete a total of 6 to 20 work/recovery periods, depending on the duration of the intervals (the shorter they are, the more you should do) and your fitness level. After completing the planned number of intervals, cool down at your warm-up effort level for five minutes. Again, more specific guidelines will come later.

Slow-and-Steady Cardio

In your modality of choice, work for 20 to 25 minutes or so at a steady, moderate intensity level (60 to 70 percent of maximum heart rate, or HR). If you don't own a heart rate monitor and don't know your maximum heart rate, you can use the talk test to find the proper intensity level. When working in the 60 to 70 percent HRmax range, you should be able to speak a complete sentence without losing your breath, but you should not be able to string multiple sentences together. In other words, you should be able to easily swear aloud about how much you hate steady-state cardio!

Low-Intensity Resistance Exercise
(Technique Practice)

Pick 8 to 12 exercises (see below for examples), and cycle through them using loads of approximately 30 percent of your estimated 1RM for these exercises. Do 15 to 20 reps per set, and keep your rest time as short as possible between sets. With each week, add a little volume (one to three total sets) until your work capacity has improved to a level you're satisfied with. Here's a basic template you can use for this type of workout:

- Dumbbell deadlift, or other hip-dominant movement
- Reverse lunge, or other single-leg movement
- Push-up, or other horizontal push movement
- Seated cable row, or other horizontal pull movement
- X-band walks, or other hip abduction movement

- Side bridge for time, or other core stability movement
- Cable triceps pressdown, or other elbow
  extension movement
- Standing cable biceps curl, or other elbow flexion movement
- Side-lying dumbbell external rotation, or other external shoulder rotation movement

Again, in Chapters 6 through 9 I will provide specific energy workout session recommendations for all three somatotypes in each phase of the Maximum Strength Program.

TRAINING STRUCTURE

Each lifting session entails a 10-minute warm-up composed of soft tissue work and mobility movements followed by 40 to 45 minutes of strength work. Very few men who lift weights do much of a warm-up before hitting the weights, and virtually no one besides team sports athletes working under the direct supervision of a strength and conditioning coach does the sort of mobility-oriented dynamic warm-ups you will do in the Maximum Strength Program. Please resist any temptation you may experience to shorten or skip these warm-ups. While you might initially feel silly doing unfamiliar movements such as the cradle walk (see page 60), and while it might at first seem unclear to you what the heck a bodyweight overhead lunge walk has to do with increasing your maximum strength, I need you to take a leap of faith, trust me, and do these things anyway. And when I ask you to do these things wearing a ballet tutu—don't question that either; just smile and nod.

Seriously, though, the dynamic warm-up exercises prepare your body for better performance and reduce injury risk by raising body temperature, lubricating the muscles and joints, and grooving appropriate movement patterns. They also increase mobility in key joints while enhancing stability in others, enabling you to perform strength movements more efficiently. In short, the dynamic warm-up helps you lift weights better, and by lifting weights better you build more strength. The tutu is for style points and convincing the ladies at the gym that you're in touch with your feminine side.

The warm-up exercises for the lower body emphasize mobility, especially for the hips. Most lifters have less than optimal hip mobility for maximal strength performance; therefore, increasing hip mobility is a major corrective objective of the Maximum Strength Program. A second objective of the warm-ups is to improve stability at the lumbar (lower) spine region, which will protect this area from injury and help you perform all of your lifts more effectively. Happily, many of the movements increase hip mobility and lumbar spine stability simultaneously.

There are only five or six strength exercises in the typical Maximum Strength Program training session, compared to as many as seven to 10 in the typical bodybuilding workout. There are two reasons behind this difference. First, in maximum strength training, there is no need to isolate individual muscle groups with the sorts of single-joint movements that are the bread and butter of bodybuilding workouts (we will use some single-joint movements for the sake of injury prevention, though). It takes a lot of different isolation movements to cover all the muscles of the upper and lower body, but it takes only a few compound, multijoint strength movements to fatigue all of the major muscle groups. They give you more bang for your buck. In addition, maximum strength exercises are performed at a very high intensity that fatigues the muscles and central nervous system relatively quickly compared to the 10RM loads that are tossed around in bodybuilding workouts.

Generally, the upper-body sessions in the Maximum Strength Program include more movements than the lower-body sessions. A greater variety of movements is necessary in training the upper body simply because it is more structurally complex than the lower body. Also, there is a need to include corrective exercises for commonly weak stabilizing muscles of the upper body such as the rotator cuff and scapular stabilizers (the muscles of your upper back and arm that stabilize the shoulder joint).

Another important difference between maximum strength training sessions and bodybuilding sessions is that, because of their higher intensity, maximum strength sessions generally require more rest time between sets. When performing sets of fewer than six reps, I recommend that you rest between sets as long as you feel is necessary to perform the next set at the same performance level as the previous one, *and then add 30 seconds.* The reason is that you will feel ready to do another set when your muscles have recovered, but your central nervous system will need a little more time. The CNS always needs more time to recover from very-high-intensity efforts than the muscles do, and it's almost impossible to assess CNS recovery by feel. On higher-rep stuff, go ahead and rest only as long as you feel is necessary to perform the next set at the same level as the previous one.

As you go through the Maximum Strength Program, you will build knowledge of your personal "recovery profile," and this knowledge will enable you to ensure optimal rest time. For example, in the early days of the program you might find that your performance plummets from set to set even though you feel you are resting long enough. By experimenting with longer rest periods, you might find that your performance improves and thereafter continue to use longer rest periods.

WORKLOAD MODULATION

The overall training workload varies from week to week within each four-week phase of the Maximum Strength Program, in the following manner:

FIRST WEEK: High workload

SECOND WEEK: Medium workload

THIRD WEEK: Very high workload

FOURTH WEEK: Low workload

One of the most common mistakes that the average weightlifter (that means *you*) makes is training at more or less the same workload every week. Varying the workload from week to week is a far more effective strategy for building strength in the long term. Cutting back the workload every other week (and especially every fourth week, in this program) enables you to train at higher intensities in the alternate weeks than you could possibly train if you hit it "all-out" every single week. A good saying to remember is that "fatigue masks fitness." The fact that you can't do something at a certain time (namely, when you've accumulated a lot of fatigue) doesn't mean that you can't do it under other circumstances (i.e., when you're rested, and you have a more pronounced psychological motivation stimulus).

The lower-workload "back-off" weeks also give your muscles greater opportunity to fulfill the adaptations triggered by the harder weeks than they would have if you kept the workload higher. The training process is all about stimulus and adaptation, but these two things don't happen simultaneously; they happen sequentially. Hard training applies the stimulus for adaptation. Subsequent lighter training facilitates adaptation and prepares the body to handle even greater stimuli.

Finally, your muscles will typically perform best at the end of a back-off week and the beginning of a week that follows a back-off week. These moments of the training process give you the opportunity to apply fully the gains you've made through recent training and recovery. Nothing stimulates future adaptations better than a training session in which you perform at your best.

FOUR PHASES

The four phases of the Maximum Strength Program are the Foundation Phase, the Build Phase, the Growth Phase, and the Peak Phase.

Phase 1: Foundation

Phase 1, or the Foundation Phase, is your introduction to maximum strength training. Think of it as a transition between the higher-volume, lower-intensity bodybuilding training to which you are probably accustomed and the hard-core heavy lifting you will do in the later phases of the Maximum Strength Program.

The training emphasis in this phase is "straight sets" in the three- to six-repetition range. The goal is to get the body accustomed to moving heavier loads than it is used to moving. The exercise selection incorporates movements with at least four distinct purposes. Some exercises are designed to strengthen typical "weak links" in the body, such as those of the posterior chain: hamstrings, glutes, and lower back. These are naturally powerful muscles that can be vital contributors to maximal lifts, but their strength is relatively underdeveloped in most lifters. In the lower-body sessions, single-leg exercises are included because they're very important for lower-extremity health and for ensuring a great functional carryover to what you do in the real world.

Other movements are designed simply to overwhelm the larger muscles and stimulate growth. There are also higher-speed exercises that serve primarily to develop efficient technique. Maximum strength lifting requires the ability to generate great force as quickly as possible (called *explosive strength*, or *rate of force development*). Most lifters are accustomed to lifting slowly; therefore, some faster lifts with lighter loads are included to develop these missing speed and efficiency elements so that they are available when the loads get really heavy later. Finally, the core exercises in this phase are mainly basic stability exercises that will lay a foundation for more advanced types of core training in later phases.

Phase 2: Build

Phase 2 is called the Build Phase because the challenging exercise selection and the higher intensity level build on the foundation established in Phase 1. The loads increase and the set length comes down, but not to the degree that they will in Phases 3 and 4. If Phase 1 was a transition between standard bodybuilding training and true maximum strength training, then Phase 2 is a transition between foundational strength training and advanced strength training.

The training emphasis in this phase is "cluster training," which entails inserting short (10-second) rest periods within straight sets, thus enabling you to lift more weight than you can in straight sets without reducing volume—or spending more time at the gym. For example, whereas in a typical straight set you might lift an 8RM load eight times and then rest, in a cluster set you would lift a heavier, 5RM load twice, then rest for 10 seconds, and then complete three more two-rep minisets with 10-second rest periods between them. In other words, in the cluster set you're lifting a 5RM load eight times in just a little more total time than it would take you to lift an 8RM load eight times in a straight set. Those short, intraset rest periods provide just enough recovery opportunity to make it possible.

Cluster training is quite challenging, yet manageable for one who's still relatively new to maximum strength training. It subjects the muscles to high levels of hypoxia (oxygen deprivation) and mechanical stress—the two key stimuli for muscle growth and strengthening. The gains you make here will help prepare your muscles to handle the extreme mechanical strain imposed by the single-rep sets over 90 percent of 1RM in Phase 4.

The pool of exercises used in this phase is larger than in Phase 1. The four weeks of Phase 1 training will have increased your neuromuscular efficiency, and the more neurally efficient you become, the more you have to rotate your exercises to stimulate additional gains. There's still an emphasis on higher-speed lifts to break you of your slow, "grind-out-every-rep" bodybuilding habits. Single-leg movements continue to predominate in lower-body sessions. The core training exercises are slightly more advanced than those in Phase 1.

Phase 3: Growth

Phase 3 is called the Growth Phase because it is the phase in which you will probably begin to see noteworthy gains in muscle size. Muscle size tends to come around more quickly when you add in a bit more volume, and in Phase 3, you'll do just that—and with heavier loading thanks to your two months of pure strength work. Ask yourself which will stimulate more muscle growth: a set of five bench presses with 225 pounds, or a set of five with 275?

The training emphasis in this phase is the stage system, which adds training volume to the existing intensity and builds more strength mainly by increasing muscle size. In the stage system you perform low-rep sets of a given movement with a heavy load and then follow up with higher-rep sets of the same movement with a slightly lighter (but still heavy) load. For example, you might do three sets of three snatch grip deadlifts followed by two sets of five reps. The slightly lighter load in the last two sets actually feels a lot lighter because of a cool neural phenomenon called *postactivation potentiation.* Simply put, this term refers to a priming effect that hard work has on the muscles, which prepares (or "potentiates") them to work even harder.

Stage-system training is a great way to increase training volume—to increase your use of the strength you've built by ratcheting up the intensity of your training previously. After four weeks of this type of training, your muscles will be good and ready to crank up the intensity again in Stage 4.

Phase 4: Peak

Phase 4 is the Peak Phase of training. The training emphasis is single-rep sets with loads greater than 90 percent of your one-rep maximum. In my opinion, this type of training is the Holy Grail of maximum strength development. It is appropriate as "peak" training because you need to build a solid foundation through other types of training before you can take full advantage of 90-plus singles, and there's no other type of training that will take your strength level any higher.

The final week of Phase 4 is a very light back-off week with one session completely eliminated to allow the body to fully recover in preparation for Moving Day. I will provide detailed guidelines for performing the four maximal lifts and jump test on Moving Day safely and optimally.

EQUIPMENT

There are several items of required gym equipment and personal gear for the Maximum Strength Program. Some of them are found only at health clubs and gyms, so a membership is an essential prerequisite for the Maximum Strength Program, unless you have one hell of a home gym setup. The equipment is as follows:

Olympic Barbells and Weights

Every gym has these things. If you train at home, make sure you have enough weights to do the 90-percent-plus singles you will do in Phase 4—when you're a lot stronger than you are today. Remember, in this program you will probably perform heavier lifts than you ever have before in your life, so the weight plates that have been adequate in your past sessions might not be adequate in the next 16 weeks, and especially in the final weeks of the program. Along these same lines, for the sake of safety, you should have a good spotter on hand to help you with handoffs on the bench press and any other lifts that justify a spotter.

Heavy Dumbbells

Everything I said above in reference to Olympic barbells and weight plates applies to dumbbells. An alternative to traditional dumbbells is "selectorized" or "quick-change" dumbbells such as the PowerBlock (www.powerblock.com), which save a lot of space by allowing the user to switch loads as easily as changing loads on a weight stack.

Squat or Power Rack

This is also standard gym equipment. Always use a safety squat rack or a rack with safety bars positioned at the appropriate height to prevent the bar from turning you into a carpet in the event of a fall.

Cable Pulley Station

A bulky, expensive piece of equipment, this one is hard to duplicate at home. You'll need a unit with high and low attachment points and the following attachments: D-handles, V-handle, and long, straight bar. Most gyms have them.

Chin-Up Bar

If you set up a chin-up bar at home, it must be sturdy enough to support your weight plus external resistance (weight plates that you will attach to the belt with a chain) for the three-rep max chin-up exercise.

Flat Bench and Fixed Incline Bench

An adjustable incline bench will do for home use.

Chest-Supported Row Station

Most gyms have this piece of equipment, but some do not. If yours doesn't, you'll have to substitute other pulling exercises for exercises requiring this piece of equipment.

External Resistance for Weighted Chin-Up

The best setup is a standard weight belt with chain attachment to which you can hook plates.

Good Shoes

The best shoe for maximum strength training has a thin heel that allows your foot to feel the ground. In other words, your shoe should closely approximate the feel of lifting barefoot. I wear Converse All-Stars. The Nike Free is also a good choice, as are wrestling shoes. A cross-trainer with some heel lift will be preferable for certain exercises requiring a high degree of ankle dorsiflexion, such as the front squat, and in your energy workouts. Thus, you will want two pairs of shoes: one pair for strength sessions and another for energy workouts.

Resistance Bands

You will need resistance bands to perform a number of mobility exercises and a few strength exercises. Most higher-end fitness clubs and chain clubs have resistance bands; many of the smaller neighborhood gyms do not. If you buy bands for home use, get two or three bands of varying resistance levels, as different resistance levels will be appropriate to different exercises. You can find them at sporting-goods and exercise equipment stores and buy them from online retailers such as Perform Better (www.PerformBetter.com). For the sake of this program, it's best to get bands without handles attached, such as Jump Stretch and Iron Woody.

Wrist Straps

Wrist wraps are accessories specially designed to help you keep a grip on the bar when lifting very heavy loads in exercises such as the deadlift. A quality leather pair costs roughly twenty dollars. A great source is APT Pro Wrist Straps (www.ProWrist-Straps.com).

Foam Roller

You will need a foam roller to do some of the mobility exercises. Foam rollers used to be found exclusively at physical therapy offices. Now they are standard equipment in many gyms and are available to purchase for home use at many exercise equipment stores and online retailers. Foam rollers come in several sizes and two shapes (cylinders and half cylinders). I recommend a three-foot cylinder. Expect to pay $8 for a basic roller and up to $35 for a more durable version (I recommend the Foam Roller Plus from www.PerformBetter.com).

Squat Box

The box squat is simply a barbell squat performed with a box underneath one's butt. The box indicates the proper depth of the squat, which is the point where the thighs come parallel to the floor. You can use a homemade box or a bench, or you can stack adjustable aerobic steps to suit your needs; just make sure your setup is nice and sturdy. There are adjustable, indestructible squat boxes designed specifically for this use, too; you can buy a squat box from an online retailer such as EliteFTS (www.elitefts.com) for approximately $180. Most gyms have something you can use for this purpose.

Chalk

Lifting chalk keeps your hands dry to give you a better grip on the bar when you're lifting heavy weights. If your gym doesn't have it, ask the manager to start supplying it, or purchase your own. Gymnastics chalk will also do the trick. If your gym doesn't allow it, it's probably a good time to start looking for a more "hard-core" gym. That said, regardless of where you're lifting, don't be messy with the chalk; clean up after yourself like a good boy.

Tape Measure

You'll need this to measure your broad jumps on Packing Day and Moving Day.

Tennis/Lacrosse Ball

You will use this when performing soft tissue work as part of the warm-up for your strength training sessions.

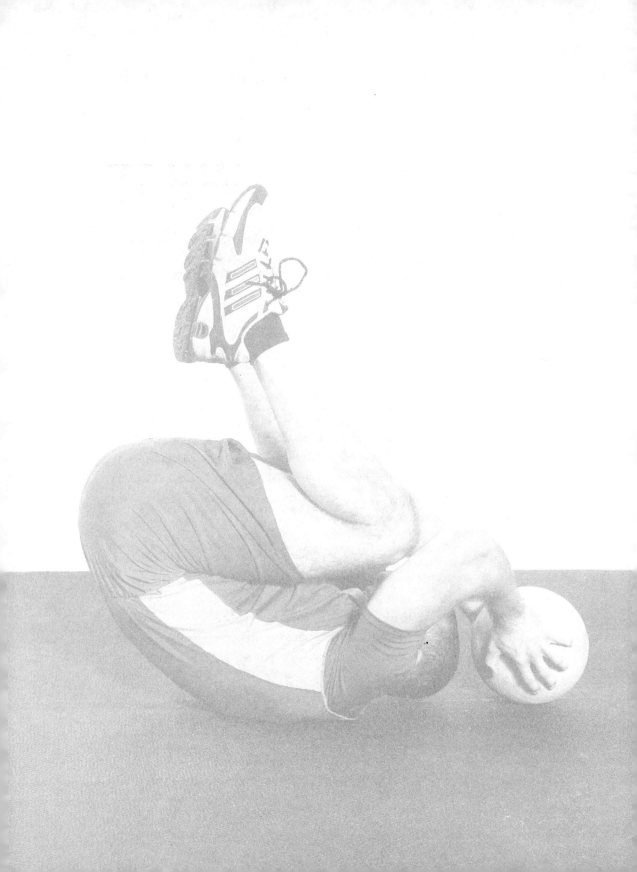

CHAPTER 4

WHAT TO EXPECT

How much stronger will I get between Packing Day and Moving Day?" I know this question is looming at the back of your mind—if not at the very front of your mind. The short answer is that only time will tell. Wait 16 weeks—or better said, *work your tail off* for 16 weeks—and you will have your answer. But as the creator of the Maximum Strength Program, I think it's only fair that I try to give you some idea of how much stronger it will make you, and also help you establish a general set of expectations for your Maximum Strength experience.

The one thing I can guarantee is that <u>if you follow the program exactly as it's written and work as hard as you can, you will get stronger.</u> How much stronger you get depends on several factors, including your past weightlifting experience, especially your training within the past few months and your genetic potential for strength improvement. Beginning weightlifters with a lot of natural strength will experience the biggest relative improvement in the five strength tests performed on Packing Day and again on Moving Day. Ectomorphs (or "hardgainers") who have already trained hard in the gym for many years will experience the smallest relative gains.

There are other factors to consider, however. One of them is the type of training you have done in the past. If your past training has involved a lot of isolation work and higher-repetition sets and little or no mobility work, soft tissue work, or muscle balance training, then you may well see huge strength improvements even if you're a grizzled gym veteran. And if injuries, sore spots, and weak links limited your strength in the past—probably due in part to a lack of mobility work, soft tissue work, and muscle balance training—then be prepared to be shocked by how much stronger you become.

The results that some of my past clients have achieved on the Maximum Strength Program will give you a more concrete sense of what to expect. A typical case is that of Doug Adams, 28, from Middle River, Maryland. Here are Doug's numbers:

	PACKING DAY	MOVING DAY
Standing Broad Jump	75.5 in.	82.5 in.
Box Squat	280 lbs.	305 lbs.
Bench Press	200 lbs.	230 lbs.
Deadlift	300 lbs.	330 lbs.
3RM Chin-Up	233 lbs.	254 lbs.

These numbers become even more impressive when you compare them to the improvements Doug was making on his own program before the Maximum Strength Program: none. Like so many recreational weightlifters, he trained consistently just to maintain the strength improvements he had achieved long ago as a beginner. If Doug had been less experienced when he started the Maximum Strength Program, the results you see in the table above would not be terribly remarkable. Even as an experienced gym goer, though, he was able to increase his maximum bench press by 15 percent in only 16 weeks, compared to no improvement in the entire preceding year, by trading his watered-down bodybuilding routine for the methods of the Maximum Strength Program.

Expect to make greater relative gains in some tests than in others. In the sport of powerlifting, nobody is equally proficient in all three lifts: the deadlift, the squat, and the bench press. Every athlete has his best lift and his worst. My strength is the deadlift. My weakness is the squat. Similarly, you may also find that you gain more proficiency in one or two of the Maximum Strength Program tests than you do in one or two others. For example, Jake Chatterton, 24, of Onslow, Iowa, improved his deadlift by a modest 15 pounds on the Maximum Strength Program, but his box squat shot up 50 pounds. Clearly, Jake had more growth potential for the squat than for the deadlift.

However, you will also tend to improve most in the movements you have least experience with. Maximum Strength Program participants typically make the smallest relative improvements in the bench press, because everybody does this exercise to death on his own, and because it's a movement where you can't move as much absolute weight compared to the squat and deadlift. Consider the example of Dan Hibbert, 34, of Calgary, Alberta, Canada. Dan made a solid 30-pound gain in his bench press (175 to 205 pounds), but his box squat skyrocketed from 165 to 245 pounds, and his deadlift jumped from 225 to 295 pounds.

The largest relative improvements almost always come in the standing broad jump, because few lifters do much power training in the gym, while the Maximum Strength Program includes plenty of it, and the standing broad jump is a pure power exercise. An extreme case is that of Mike Czobit, 22, of Mississauga, Ontario. Mike's standing broad jump was only 42 inches on Packing Day. Sixteen weeks later, on Moving Day, he leaped 78 inches. That's an 86 percent increase!

The greater your overall commitment to getting stronger, the bigger your gains will be. A case in point is Chris Paul, 31, of Danbury, Connecticut. Already an experienced lifter going into the Maximum Strength Program, Chris made a total lifestyle commitment to getting stronger and put some very impressive results on the board even though the fourth-month program coincided with the busiest period in the history of his business:

	PACKING DAY	MOVING DAY
Standing Long Jump	91.5 in.	97.5 in.
1 RM Box Squat	315 lbs.	395 lbs.
1 RM Bench Press	265 lbs.	295 lbs.
1 RM Deadlift	385 lbs.	435 lbs.
3RM Chin-Up	196 lbs. + 45 lbs.	196 + 55 lbs.
Body Weight	190 lbs.	195 lbs.

What could have possibly played into Chris's superior results? A few potential explanations are training environment (he trained at a hard-core gym surrounded by strong guys who pushed him all the way through the program), nutrition (Chris is very on point with his nutrition), sheer effort, and sleep quality. The take-home message from Chris's

EARLIER BEDTIMES + ZMA.

results is that there are a lot of other factors to which you need to attend in order to make *optimal* progress instead of just *good* progress.

On the general topic of what to expect from the Maximum Strength Program, but beyond the specific topic of strength gains, you should also be prepared to notice some significant changes in the size, shape, and composition of your body. The majority of Maximum Strength Program participants gain weight, because it's hard to gain a ton of strength without also significantly increasing your muscle mass. Among those who do gain weight, the average amount of weight gain is approximately seven pounds. This weight gain is usually accounted for entirely by muscle growth. In fact, body fat measurements indicate that Maximum Strength Program participants frequently gain more muscle weight than they do body weight; that is, they lose fat simultaneously.

Those who start the Maximum Strength Program with the goal of losing weight while gaining strength invariably do so by following the program's nutrition guidelines and taking advantage of the flexibility of its energy workout prescriptions. For example, Ryan Gleason, 24, of Derby, Connecticut, dropped from 244 to 237 pounds on the Maximum Strength Program and reduced his body fat percentage from 23 percent to 19 percent, while greatly increasing his strength.

Other important results you can expect to get from the Maximum Strength Program are less quantifiable. These include improvements in posture, mobility, sports performance, and enjoyment of weightlifting along with less susceptability to injury. Ryan Gleason, whom I just mentioned above, reported, "The program's mix of mobility and soft tissue work has enabled me to overcome all of my old injuries." That's one I hear all the time. You may even experience surprising benefits that go beyond the gym. "The Maximum Strength Program changed my life," Preston Oliver, 23, of Glastonbury, Connecticut, told me. "It gave me the knowledge to radically change my body, increase my strength, and improve my health. It also gave me confidence and motivation to use these tools and better myself in all aspects of my life."

The final aspect of the Maximum Strength Program experience that I would like to prepare you for is completely different. Up to this point I have been talking about the results you can expect to achieve. Now I wish to state explicitly what you must be prepared to do to get these results: work hard! Most Maximum Strength Program graduates report that they have never worked harder in the gym. Jake Chatterton put it this way: "Certainly, not every session was what most people would call 'fun.' This isn't

one of those programs where you can admire yourself in front of the mirror while doing endless sets of arm curls. This program was tough. It was exhausting at times, both
physically and mentally. But the testing day at the end of the program was where the
dividends were paid."

Keep these words in mind when you experience your own tough days—and weeks—on
the Maximum Strength Program. Hang in there, and the dividends will be paid!

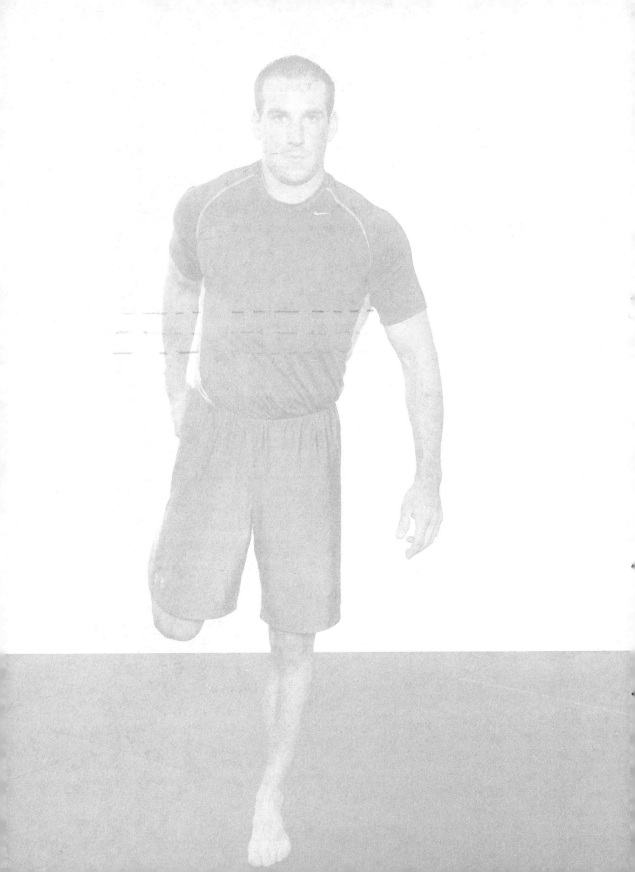

CHAPTER 5

MAXIMUM STRENGTH WARM-UPS

I know how it must feel to be a dentist. All day long dentists ask their patients how often they floss their teeth, only to learn what they already know (that the patients seldom or never floss), and then urge their patients to start doing it daily, as it would spare them the pain of the drill.

Similarly, I spend time almost every day urging clients and others to do soft tissue exercises and mobility work consistently to warm up for training sessions. Most lifters avoid this type of stuff because they feel pressed for time in the gym, and they want to go straight to the iron. I try to coax guys out of this mind-set by explaining that they will get better results in the *long run* if they spend the same amount of time in the gym, but make time for thorough warm-ups. Soft tissue work and mobility exercises improve the basic health of the musculoskeletal system, improving posture, mobility, lifting technique, and performance, and reducing injuries. These techniques give you a more solid foundation to build on with your lifting, enabling you to build a bigger, stronger structure over time.

The advantage that I have over dentists is that they see their patients only twice a year, whereas I see my clients once a week at least. I can more or less force them to give my warm-ups a try, and in almost every case they are so pleased with the results that they happily continue doing them on their own. Unfortunately, I can't track you down at your gym to make you do the soft tissue work and mobility warm-ups that are an essential and mandatory part of every Maximum Strength Program training session, but I urge you to take a leap of faith and perform them with an open mind. After 16 weeks your body will feel so balanced and sound, you wouldn't stop doing the warm-ups if I paid you.

Each warm-up takes 10 to 15 minutes to complete. It begins with 10 soft tissue manipulations that involve either a foam roller or a tennis ball. Then you move on to do 11 different mobility exercises. By the time you complete these exercises your body will be primed to perform optimally on your subsequent lifts. And as the days and weeks go by, you will see and feel your posture, mobility, technique, and overall musculoskeletal health improve.

There are two versions of the Maximum Strength Program warm-up. Both include the same set of 10 soft tissue manipulations, but they include different mobility exercises. In this chapter, I will present first all of the soft tissue manipulations and mobility exercises. A table at the end of the chapter lays out the details of the two versions of the warm-up.

SOFT TISSUE WORK

Everyone knows that muscles need to be pliable and stretchable in order to function properly and enable us to carry out the movements we face both in sports and our everyday lives, but very few people pay attention to the *quality* of their muscle tissue. The soft tissue work outlined in the next few pages will likely be a bit uncomfortable at first, but you'll feel like a million bucks as you start to clear up those knots and trigger points in muscles throughout your body as well as adhesions in connective tissues. Foam rolling and lacrosse/tennis ball work are like having the world's cheapest massage therapist; you'll be amazed by how quickly a little rolling can improve the quality of your movement and how you feel.

You'll want to spend about 15 to 20 seconds on each spot—and possibly a little more time on the areas that feel the most "knotted up." Perform all of the movements described in the following pages at a very slow pace.

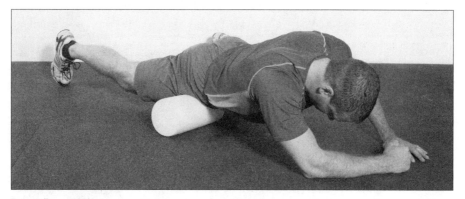

Foam Roller — Hip Flexors

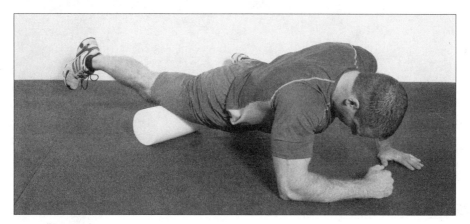

Foam Roller — Quadriceps

FOAM ROLLER

The following soft tissue manipulations require the use of a foam roller.

Hip Flexors

Set up on your forearms with the top of one thigh on the roller. Slowly roll back and forth from the upper thigh up to the crest of the hip, stopping short of the prominent aspect of your pelvis.

Quadriceps

Set up as you would for the hip flexor manipulation. This manipulation is quite similar to the hip flexor manipulation, but you'll just work your way down further on the thigh—right down to the point at which the quadricep meets the kneecap.

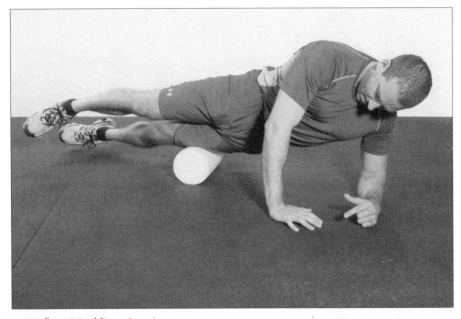

Foam Roller — IT Band/Tensor Fascia Latae

IT Band/Tensor Fasciae Latae

This is unquestionably the most uncomfortable (yet beneficial) manipulation of the bunch. It loosens the IT band, which is the large tendon running along the outer side of the thigh, and the tensor fascia latae, which is the large muscle attached to the IT band. Lie crosswise like a human teeter-totter on the foam roller, which should be positioned underneath your outer thigh about an inch below the hip bone. Use the forearm of your downside arm and the hand of your topside arm to pull your body forward so that your outer thigh slides across the foam roller all the way down to the kneecap. It may sound silly, but imagine trying to pull the quad off the bone. (That's certainly what it will feel as if you're doing.) Now slide back in the opposite direction. You should just be able to complete two back-and-forth slides in 20 seconds.

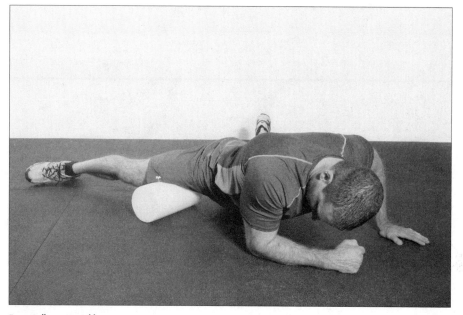

Foam Roller — Hip Adductors

Hip Adductors

Lie face down on the floor with your hips opened up, so your inner thighs face the floor. Begin with the foam roller pinned between the upper inner thigh of one leg and the floor. Pull your body along the floor with your forearms to slide your inner thigh over the foam roller from just short of the groin all the way down to the inside of the knee. Most people notice some restrictions just above the knee. Now slide back in the other direction. You should just be able to complete two back-and-forth slides in 20 seconds.

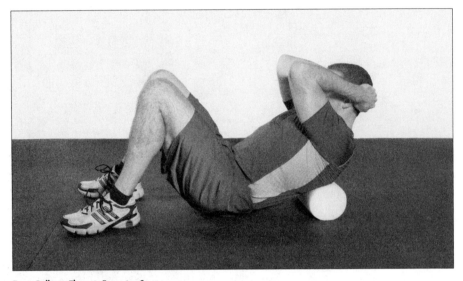

Foam Roller — Thoracic Extension Start

Thoracic Extension

The foam roller thoracic extension isn't a traditional foam rolling movement, as it isn't intended to loosen up knots in muscle tissue. Rather, the roller acts as a "hinge" that helps you improve your thoracic-spine-extension range of motion.

Sit on the floor with the roller behind you, positioned perpendicular to your body. Keeping your butt and feet on the floor, ease back to the roller so that it's positioned about an inch below the base of your shoulder blades. Lightly grab the back of your head with your hands, and pull the elbows together. Keeping your chin tucked, extend back as if you were trying

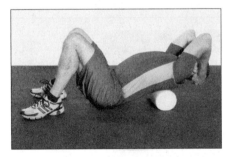

Foam Roller — Thoracic Extension Finish

to touch the back of your head to the floor. All the range of motion should come at the middle and upper back. After a pause in the bottom position, return to the top position, and then slide the roller a bit higher up on your upper back and repeat.

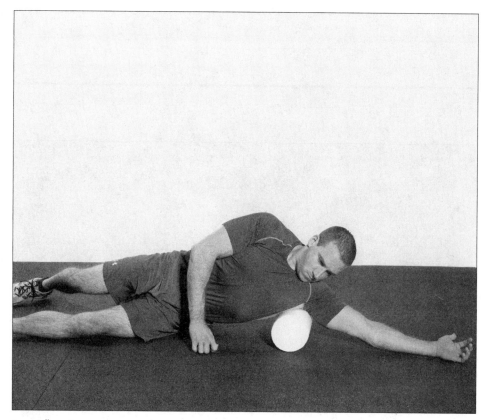

Foam Roller — Lats

Lats

Lie on your side with the roller positioned perpendicular to your body and "jammed" in your armpit, with your arm extended as though you're swimming the sidestroke.

Roll from the point where the lat attaches to the upper arm all the way down to the base of the shoulder blade.

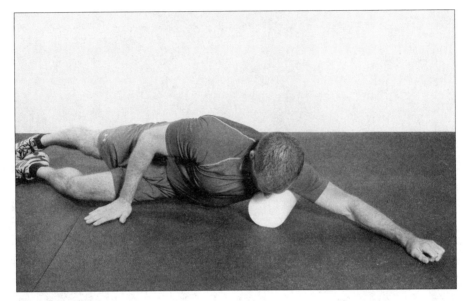

Foam Roller—Pecs

Pecs

Imagine your body is a clock face with your head at the 12 o'clock position. Raise your left arm out to <u>10 o'clock</u> and lie facedown with the roller positioned perpendicular to your arm and your left pec resting on it. Roll your pec over the foam roller from the pec attachment on the upper arm down to about where your nipple is. Repeat this manipulation with your right arm in the <u>2 o'clock</u> position.

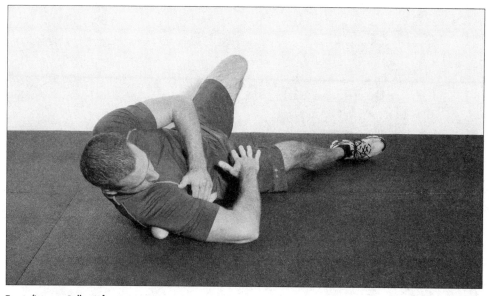

Tennis/Lacrosse Ball — Infraspinatus Start

TENNIS/LACROSSE BALL

The following soft tissue manipulations require the use of a tennis or lacrosse ball.

Infraspinatus

Lie on your side with the ball pinned between the floor and the back side of your shoulder near your armpit (it'll feel like the attachment of the lats, but it's actually a muscle called the *infraspinatus*). Use small movements to knead the flesh in this area. You'll likely notice quite a few "hot spots," and when you do, bear down on them a bit, and gradually move your arm through internal and external rotation to loosen them up.

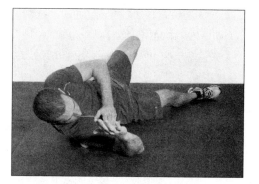

Tennis/Lacrosse Ball — Infraspinatus Finish

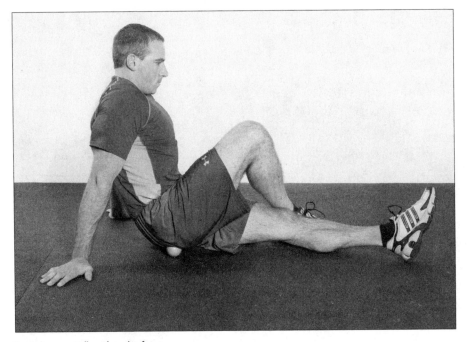

Tennis/Lacrosse Ball — Glutes/Piriformis

Glutes/Piriformis

This one will be a pain in your butt, both literally and figuratively! To work on the right glutes/piriformis (a buttock muscle that externally rotates the thigh), sit on the ball with your right cheek and cross your right leg over your left. Start by working on the outside portion of the glutes, and then move upward and toward the midline to get the piriformis a bit more.

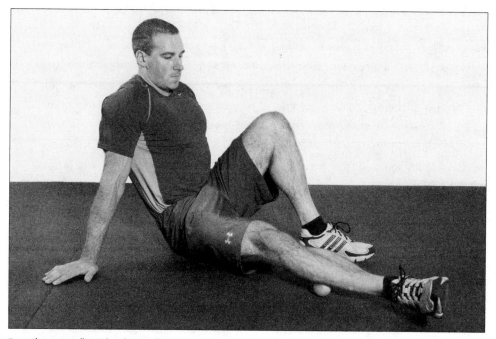

Tennis/Lacrosse Ball — Calves/Peroneals

Calves/Peroneals

To roll out the calf muscles and peroneal muscles (which run along the outside of the shin), simply sit on the floor with the ball underneath one calf, apply some of your body weight to the ball, and knead the tissue by moving the calf up and down and side to side over the ball. You'll want to hit three spots: inside, outside, and down by the Achilles tendon.

MOBILITY EXERCISES

You don't need a gymnast's flexibility to increase your maximal strength performance. But you do need the ability to move your joints through a normal range of motion with stability, control, and efficiency. In other words, you need a certain degree of mobility. These exercises will give you the mobility you need to increase your maximal strength safely and productively.

The great thing about them is that they have both acute and cumulative benefits. Not only will they improve the way your joints move over time, but they will also produce small, immediate improvements that will enable you to perform better in each weightlifting session. That's why they're done as a warm-up!

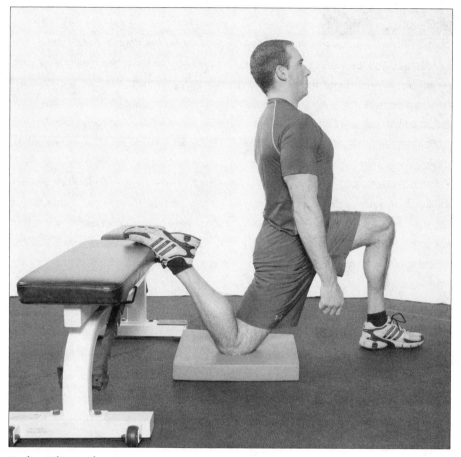

Kneeling RF/TFL Stretch

Kneeling RF/TFL Stretch

BENEFITS: This two-part stretch loosens up the rectus femoris and tensor fascia latae, two of the hip flexors that are commonly tight.

ACTION: Kneel in a lunge position. Without moving the back knee from the floor, take the foot of the back leg and place it on a bench behind you. Push the hip of the same leg forward and tighten up your glutes. After 10 seconds, rotate at the hips slightly in the direction of the front leg and hold the stretch for 10 seconds more. Repeat the stretch on the opposite side. Feel free to put a towel or pad on the floor under your knee for comfort.

Sleeper Stretch

BENEFITS: This stretch is aimed at improving the internal rotation range of motion at the upper arm. Stiffness in the rear of the shoulder girdle (the area around the shoulder blades) is often the culprit in shoulder problems, and this stretch has proven highly effective in helping to correct that problem.

ACTION: Lie on your side with your bottom-side shoulder blade "jammed" underneath you to hold it in place. Imagine pushing the chest out to ensure that the shoulder blade is held back and down. Your bottom-side arm should begin in an arm-wrestling position on the floor, with the upper arm at a right angle to your body and your forearm pointing toward the ceiling.

Using your top-side hand, lightly push your bottom-side wrist toward the floor to create an internal rotation movement at your shoulder (as though you're winning your arm-wrestling match). When this action is performed correctly, you'll feel a stretch along the back side of the bottom shoulder. This should be a *gentle* stretch; on a scale of 0 to 10, it should be only a 3 or 4. Hold for 15 seconds.

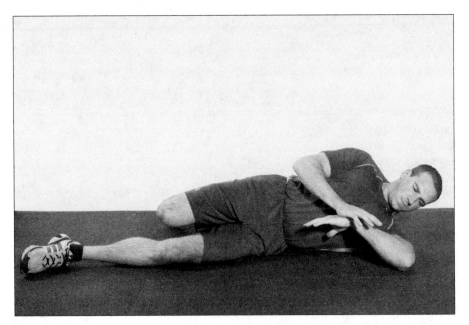

Sleeper Stretch

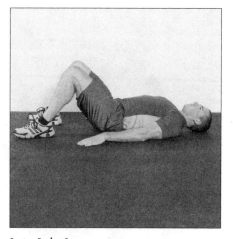

Supine Bridge Start

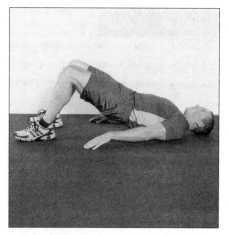

Supine Bridge Finish

Supine Bridge

BENEFITS: The supine bridge is a very basic exercise designed to activate the glutes.

ACTION: Lie on your back with your legs bent to approximately 90 degrees and your feet flat on the floor. Squeeze your glutes as if you're trying to pinch a quarter between them, and pop your hips up in the air. Hold and squeeze at the top of this movement, then return under control to the starting position. Make sure that you do not hyperextend your lumbar (lower) spine. If you feel the movement in your back, you're performing it incorrectly. Do your best to minimize hamstring involvement. A good trick for reducing the hamstrings' contribution is to lightly touch the quadriceps with your hands during the set (if the quads are activated, the hamstrings have to relax a bit). Perform one set of 12 repetitions.

Reach, Roll, and Lift

BENEFITS: I picked up this drill from Mike Robertson and Bill Hartman in their Inside-Out DVD, and it instantly became one of my favorites for activating the lower trapezius, a muscle that's very important in upward rotation of the shoulder blade.

ACTION: Kneel on the floor and position your forearms on the floor with your elbows in close to your knees. Lift one arm and extend it straight forward without lifting the head. Roll the hand so that the palm faces up, and then lift it up by driving through your shoulder blade (keep the elbow extended). When this movement is performed correctly, you'll feel it closer to your mid back. Most people will note that they have more range of motion on the side of their dominant arm. Perform eight repetitions on each side.

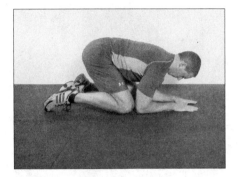

Reach, Roll, and Lift Start

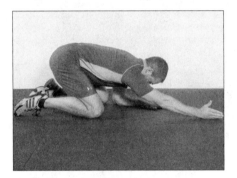

Reach, Roll, and Lift Middle

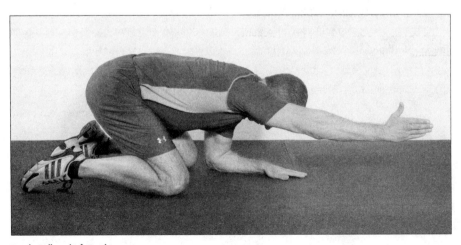

Reach, Roll, and Lift Finish

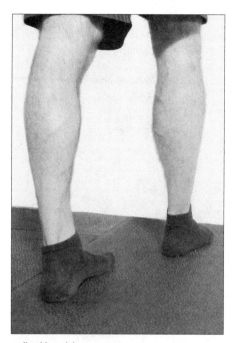 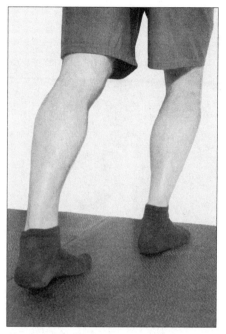

Wall Ankle Mobilization Start   Wall Ankle Mobilization Finish

Wall Ankle Mobilization

BENEFITS: This mobility drill increases range of motion in dorsiflexion (pulling the toes of the foot toward the shin), a component of ankle mobility that most people lack nowadays, thanks to high heels, shoes and boots with big heels and strong lateral supports, and ankle-taping in sports.

ACTION: Stand facing a wall, with the toes of one foot against the wall, and break the knee forward to tap the wall with your kneecap. Now slide the foot back a bit so that your toes are about an inch away from the wall, and repeat. Keep moving back little by little until you get to the exact point where the kneecap is *barely* touching the wall. Make sure that your knee goes straight forward and not inward (knock-knee), and that the heel remains on the floor the entire time. Perform eight repetitions on each side.

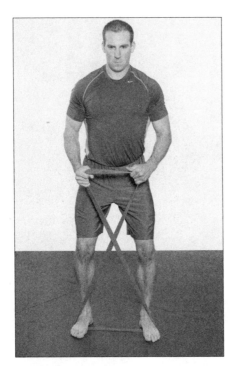

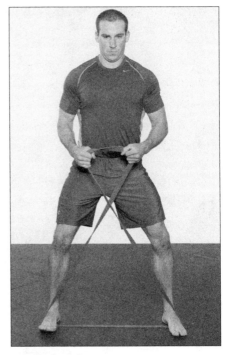

X-Band Walk Start   **X-Band Walk Finish**

X-Band Walk

BENEFITS: The X-band walk, the clever creation of strength coach Mike Boyle, is a great exercise for activating the gluteus medius (a buttock muscle that rotates the hip outward), which is very important for knee and hip health.

ACTION: Loop a half-inch or 1-inch band under both feet and stand on top of it. Your feet should be roughly 12 inches apart at the start. Cross the ends of the band to form an *X* and grasp one end in each hand, pulling the ends taut. Lift your chest up and shoulders back, and keep tension on the band throughout.

Start walking sideways with small lateral steps. The leg that's on the side of the direction you're moving will have to overcome the band's tension to take each step. Make sure that you keep the hips and shoulders level, and don't deviate forward or backward as you go to the side. When this exercise is performed correctly, you'll feel the movement in your glutes. Complete 10 steps in one direction and then 10 more moving in the opposite direction.

Pull-Back Butt Kick

BENEFITS: This exercise works to lengthen the quadriceps and hip flexor muscles.

ACTION: From a standing position, take a step forward and kick the heel of one leg backward toward your glutes. Using the hand on the same side, actively pull the heel into your glutes and come up on the toes of the opposite foot simultaneously. Maintain good posture (avoid forward leaning), and do not allow the leg to move too far to the side. Hold this position for a count of "one-one-thousand," and then place your foot back on the floor and repeat this movement with the opposite leg. Perform five repetitions with each leg.

Those who are really tight will try to lean forward and/or move the leg out to the side to grab the foot. These actions are compensations for a lack of range of motion in hip extension and should be avoided.

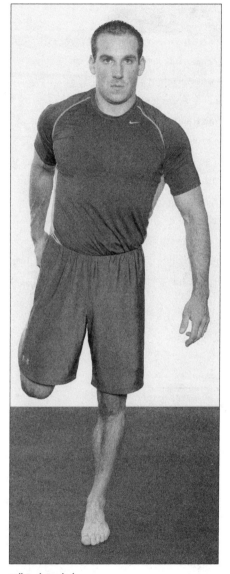

Pull-Back Buttkick

Cradle Walk

BENEFITS: This mobility drill works to increase hip external-rotation range of motion.

ACTION: From a standing position, step forward and pull the instep of the nonsupporting leg upward with both hands. The knee will bend and the hip will externally rotate. Maintain good posture and actively pull the foot up rather than just grasping it. Don't round the shoulders in the process; bring the leg toward the upper body and not vice versa. Perform five repetitions on each side.

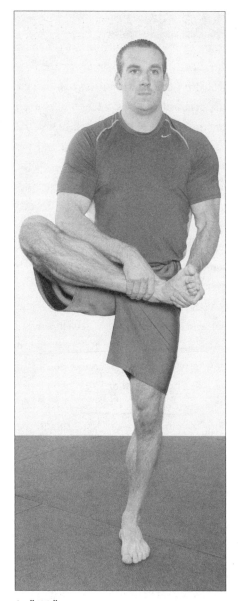

Cradle Walk

Split-Stance Broomstick Pec Mobilization

BENEFITS: This is another drill I learned from Indianapolis-based physical therapist Bill Hartman. It not only loosens up the pectoral muscles, but it also (albeit indirectly) helps to coordinate the neuromuscular link between the shoulder and the opposite hip and ankle.

ACTION: Stand with your feet in a split stance with the right foot 18 to 24 inches behind the left (depending on your level of flexibility). Make sure that the toes on both feet are pointed straight ahead, and that the heels of both feet are on the ground. Hold the end of a broomstick or any similar object out in front of you with the left end in the palm of your left hand and the midpoint of the broomstick in your right hand with an overhand grip.

Imagine your body is a clock face with the head at the 12 o'clock position. Use your right hand to push the broomstick and with it your left arm back to 10 o'clock. When you feel a good stretch in your left pec, return to the starting position and repeat. Make sure that you don't rotate at your torso or allow the feet to pivot. The most common error in performing this exercise is external rotation of the back leg. Perform eight repetitions on each side.

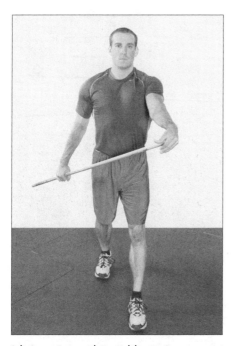

Split-Stance Broomstick Pec Mobilization Start

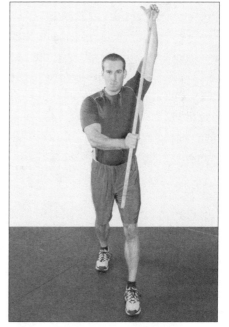

Split-Stance Broomstick Pec Mobilization Finish

Squat to Stand

BENEFITS: This is an excellent drill for mobilizing the hamstrings and inner thighs and for helping those with mobility deficits squat deeper.

ACTION: Stand with your feet positioned slightly farther than a shoulder width apart. Bend over and grab the bottoms of your toes with your hands, bending your knees as much as necessary to do so. From here, use your arms to pull yourself into a deep squat position. Try to keep the chest up, the knees out, and a slight arch in the lower back. Hold for a second or two in the "hole" before standing up and repeating the movement.

The goal is to get a little lower with a little bit better posture with each repetition. All of the technique elements that are important in a regular squat are important here. Most importantly, you want to keep ideal posture with the chest up and the back flat. Also, don't let your heels rise up in the bottom position. Perform one set of eight repetitions.

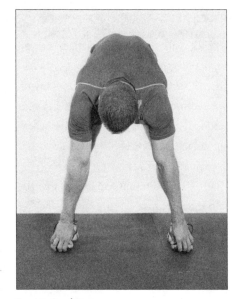

Squat-to-Stand Start

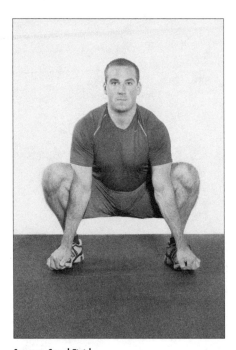

Squat-to-Stand Finish

Overhead Lunge Walk

BENEFITS: This movement mobilizes the hip flexors and improves single-leg stability.

ACTION: Stand normally and raise both arms straight overhead. Take a long step forward with one leg, and bend both knees until the knee of the trailing leg grazes the floor. Thrust forward off the front foot, and take a lunge with the opposite leg, keeping your arms raised. The front heel should remain in contact with the floor on each stride. Perform five repetitions on each side.

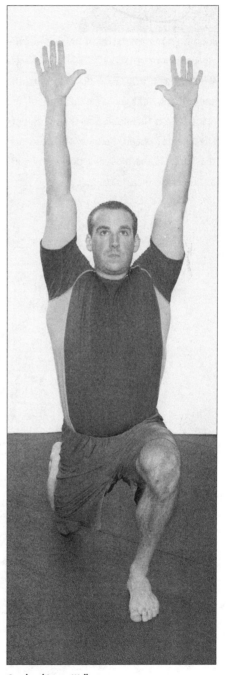

Overhead Lunge Walk

Warrior Lunge Stretch

BENEFITS: This basic stretch loosens up the hip flexors.

ACTION: Kneel in a lunge position with the knee of the rear leg and the foot of the front leg on the floor and the arms outstretched overhead. Keeping the head and chest up, let the hips sink down and shift your weight forward so you get a stretch in the front of the hip of the leg whose knee is in contact with the floor. Don't place your hands on your knee or lean too far forward or arch the back to increase the stretch; just let the hips sink and shift forward. Hold for 15 seconds and then switch sides.

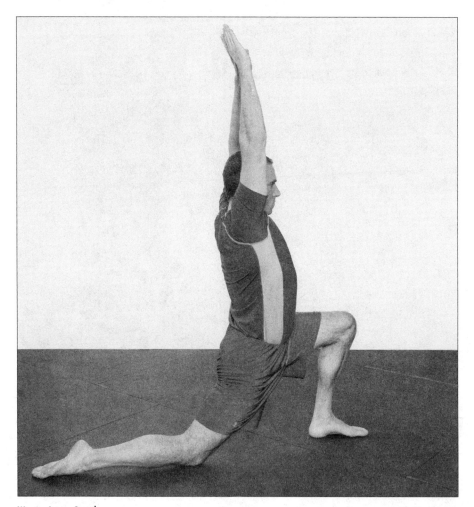

Warrior Lunge Stretch

Seated 90/90 Stretch

BENEFITS: This stretch is aimed at improving hip external-rotation range of motion.

ACTION: While seated on a chair or bench, cross the right leg over the left so that the outside of the right ankle is in contact with the left lower thigh. With your left hand, pull the right instep up toward your face while pushing the right knee/shin downward with your right hand. You should feel a stretch along the outside of the right thigh right where it meets the glutes. Hold the stretch 15 seconds and relax. Reverse your position and stretch the left side.

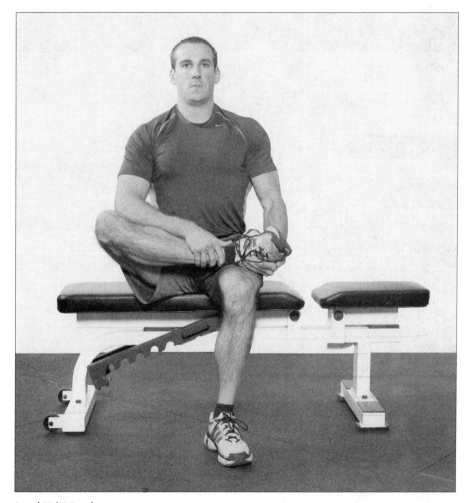

Seated 90/90 Stretch

+ Pistol Squats in warmup

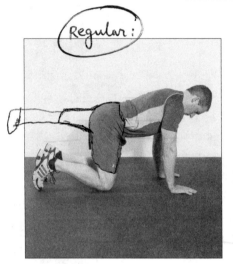

Regular:

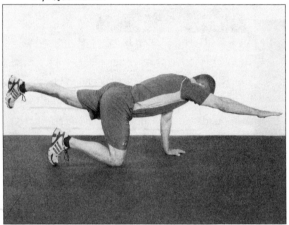

Advanced:

Bird Dog Start   **Bird Dog Finish**

Bird Dog

BENEFITS: Popularized by Dr. Stuart McGill as a premier lower-back rehabilitation movement, the bird dog is an excellent exercise for improving strength and motor control in the glutes and also for developing the stabilizing muscles in the back.

ACTION: Start on all fours, with the knees under the hips and palms under the shoulders. Look straight down at the floor with the chin tucked. Brace the stomach (as if protecting yourself from a punch), squeeze the glutes, and lift one leg and extend it straight backward in line with your torso.

Hold this position for two seconds and then return to the starting position, but with the knee hovering just above the ground (not resting on it). Make sure you keep your glute active and stomach tight throughout this exercise. This way, you will keep the hips square and steady, thus maintaining the focus on the glutes.

Once you've mastered the leg movement, you may increase the challenge level of the exercise by extending the opposite arm straight forward in line with your torso as you extend your leg. The goal is to keep everything tight and the hips steady throughout. Make sure to use your muscles and not momentum to complete the reps! Do eight repetitions on each side.

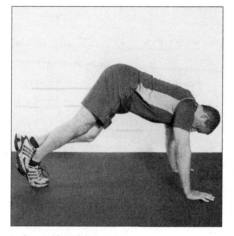

Rocking Ankle Mobilization Start

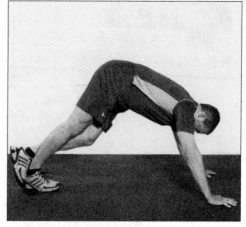

Rocking Ankle Mobilization Finish

Switch sides every other rep ("one-one thousand")
Bend knee to get more Soleus
Straight leg to get more Gastrocnemius

Rocking Ankle Mobilization

BENEFITS: This is an excellent movement for warming up the calves and improving ankle mobility—a very common deficit that can lead to a host of injuries and conditions such as knee pain, shin splints, and plantar fasciitis.

ACTION: Start in the "pike" position with the palms and toes of both feet on the floor, the arms and legs straight, and the hips up higher than the rest of the body. Place the left foot against the right Achilles tendon and press the heel of the right foot down to the floor, holding at the bottom position for a count of "one-one-thousand." Reverse your position and stretch the left side. You can also perform repetitions with the knee slightly bent to change the emphasis to the soleus (the inner calf muscle) instead of the gastrocnemius (the outer calf muscle). Perform eight repetitions on each side.

Scapular Push-Up

BENEFITS: The scapular push-up strengthens the serratus anterior, a muscle that essentially holds the shoulder blade tight to the rib cage to prevent scapular winging. It's a crucial muscle for optimal shoulder stability.

ACTION: Assume a standard push-up position at the top. Keeping your elbows locked, retract the shoulder blades so that your torso sinks a couple of inches toward the floor. Keep your elbows locked. Now protract your shoulder blades fully, so that your upper back takes on a slightly hunched look. Keep your elbows locked. Finally, return to the starting position. Did I mention to keep your elbows locked? Perform 12 repetitions.

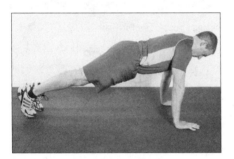

Scapular Push-Up Start and Finish (Shoulder Blades Protracted)

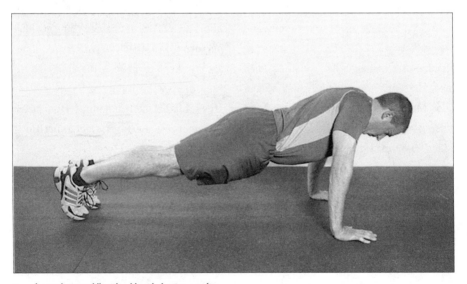

Scapular Push-Up Middle (Shoulder Blades Retracted)

Scapular Wall Slide

BENEFITS: This exercise is another variation to strengthen the lower trapezius to keep your shoulders healthy during upward rotation.

ACTION: Stand with your upper back and butt against a wall. Walk your feet out approximately 18 inches away from the wall. Lift both arms overhead and hold them back against the wall behind you.

From the starting position, try to pull your elbows back into the wall and down. Do your best to keep the back flat; a flat back will give the rib cage an outwardly protruding appearance. Keep the elbows on the wall and the hands as close to the wall as possible (those with really poor flexibility won't be able to get the hands to the wall). Also keep your head back against the wall for the duration of the set. If this exercise is performed correctly with the chin tucked, you'll look as if you have a "double chin" for the entire set! Squeeze your shoulder blades down in the bottom position for a count of "one-one-thousand." Perform 12 repetitions.

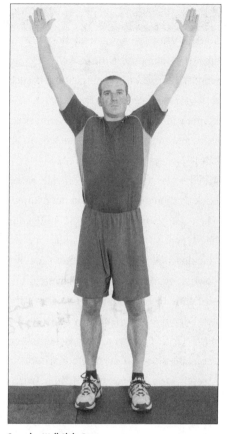

Scapular Wall Slide Start

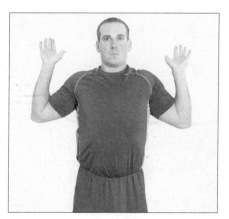

Scapular Wall Slide Finish

Levator Scapulae/Upper Trap Stretch

BENEFITS: With the amount of time people spend at computers nowadays, it's no wonder the forward head posture is such a widespread problem. This stretch will help to loosen up some of the muscles that are most commonly locked up in "desk jockeys."

ACTION: Place your left hand on your lower back as though you are being handcuffed. Then use your right hand to pull your head gently to the right and forward (tucking the chin) so that you're looking down at your right foot. The secret to this stretch is to make sure that you keep the shoulder blade pulled down so that the posterior and lateral neck musculature on the right side will stretch out. Hold the stretch for 15 seconds and then switch sides.

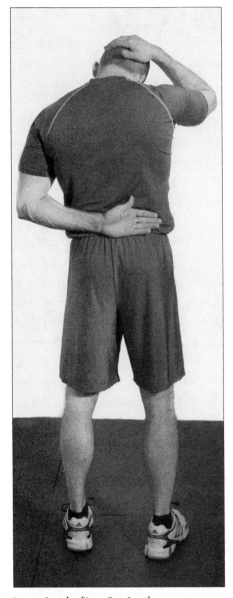

Levator Scapulae/Upper Trap Stretch

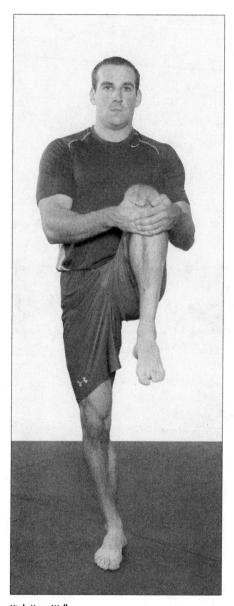

High-Knee Walk

High-Knee Walk

BENEFITS: This mobility drill is great for getting range of motion in the glutes and hamstrings while working to improve your balance and coordination as well.

ACTION: From a standing position, bend your left leg and lift your left knee as high as you can. Actively pull the knee up and toward your chest with both hands, and <u>come up on the toes of the opposite foot</u>, holding this position for a count of "one-one-thousand." Maintain good posture, <u>avoiding forward lean</u>, and keep the <u>chin tucked.</u> Release the left knee and place the left foot down a step ahead of the right. Now take a high-knee step with the right leg. Perform five repetitions on each side.

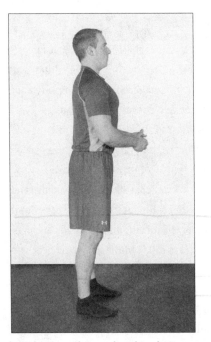

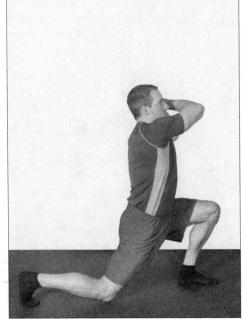

Reverse Lunge with Posterolateral Reach Start   Reverse Lunge with Posterolateral Reach Finish

Reverse Lunge with Posterolateral Reach

BENEFITS: This is another great exercise I picked up from Robertson and Hartman in their *Inside-Out* DVD. It works to loosen up tight hip flexors while enhancing range of motion at the opposite shoulder. Believe it or not, there is a critical functional link between one shoulder and the opposite hip and ankle.

Cosgrove said that on T-Nation too,

ACTION: Begin in a standing position with your hands clasped together and your arms extended toward the floor in front of you. Take a long stride backward into a lunge, and sink down until your trailing knee grazes the floor. As you step back, while keeping your hands clasped together, reach across the shoulder that's opposite the lunging leg as if you are throwing a shovelful of dirt over your shoulder. Drive off the front heel to return to starting position. Keep the chest up throughout the movement. Perform five repetitions with the left leg lunging back, and then five more with the right leg lunging back.

Walking Spiderman

BENEFITS: This movement mobilizes the inner thigh and hip flexors, making it a great "bang for your buck" warm-up movement.

ACTION: From a standing position, take a long stride forward and slightly out to the side and sink into a deep lunge position. Place both hands flat on the floor beneath your shoulders. From this position, drive off the forward foot, return to the upright position, and pull your trailing leg even with your forward leg. Repeat the movement with the opposite leg. Continue lunging forward in a walking manner. Keep the chest up and try not to let the lower back round as you lunge. A slight rounding of the upper back is OK, but don't let it get out of hand. The deeper you go with your lunges, the better the stretch will be for your inner thighs, so be sure to take long strides. Perform five repetitions on each side.

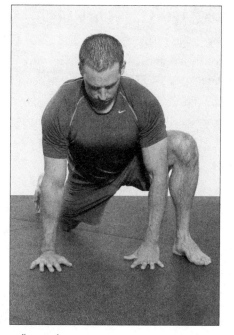

Walking Spiderman

MAXIMUM STRENGTH WARM-UP ROUTINES

The table on the opposite page presents the two complete Maximum Strength Program warm-ups. Always perform one of them in its entirety before each weightlifting session. You may either alternate consistently between the two or do whichever one you most feel like doing on a given day.

NOTE: Do all warm-ups barefoot, if possible.

CHEDULE

	WARM-UP OPTION 2

FOAM ROLLING:

- IT Band/Tensor Fasciae Latae ✓
- Quads ✓
- Hip Flexors ✓
- Hip Adductors ✓
- Thoracic Extension ✓
- Pecs — *Out (FH)* ✗
- Lats ✓

FOAM ROLLING:

- IT Band/Tensor Fasciae Latae
- Quads
- Hip Flexors
- Hip Adductors
- Thoracic Extension
- Pecs
- Lats

TENNIS/LACROSSE BALL:

- Calves/Peroneals *(Inside/outside/Achilles)* ✓
- Glutes/Piriformis ✓
- Infraspinatus ✓

TENNIS/LACROSSE BALL:

- Calves/Peroneals
- Glutes/Piriformis
- Infraspinatus

Kneeling RF / TFL Stretch	15s /side		Warrior Lunge Stretch	15s /side
Sleeper Stretch	15s /side		Seated 90/90 Stretch	15s /side
Supine Bridge *(Hip thrusts squeeze quarter b/t glutes)*	1x12		Bird Dog	8/side
Reach, Roll, and Lift	8/side		X-Band Walk	10/side
~~Wall Ankle Mobilization~~ → ✗ ✗ ✗	~~8/side~~		Rocking Ankle Mobilization	8/side
X-Band Walk	10/side		Scapular Push-Up	1x12
Pull-Back Butt Kick	5/side		Scapular Wall Slide	1x12
Cradle Walk	5/side		Levator Scapulae/Upper Trap Stretch	15s /side
Split-Stance Broomstick Pec Mobilization *OR Woodchoppers w/Pec stretch*	8/side		High-Knee Walk	5/side
Squat-to-Stand	1x8		Reverse Lunge w/Posterolateral Reach *(shovelling dirt)*	5/side
Overhead Lunge Walk	5/side		Walking Spiderman	5/side

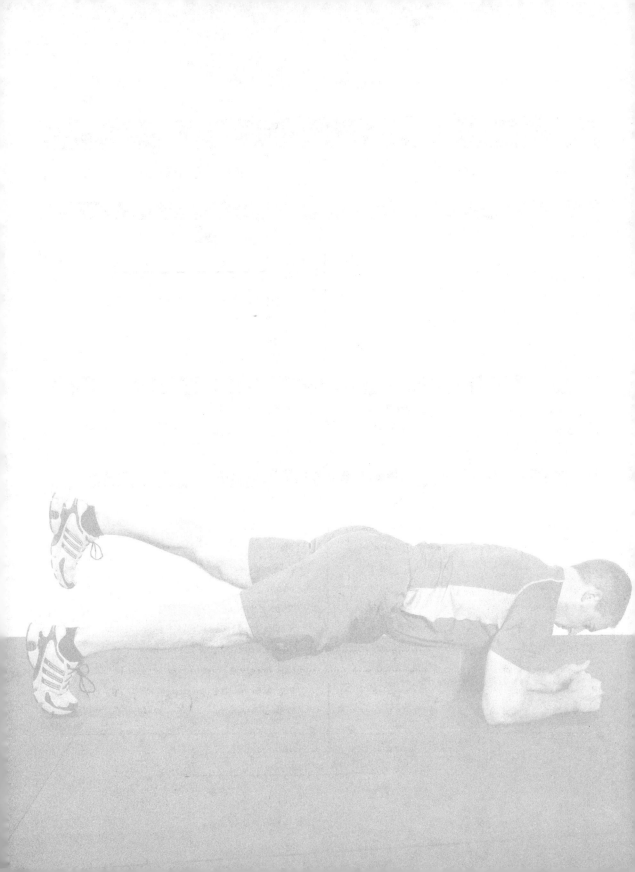

CHAPTER 6

PHASE 1: FOUNDATION

E nough chit chat. It's time to start the Maximum
Strength Program. Step 1 is to do your pretesting.
Follow the pretesting instructions presented in
the next section, and record your results on the table
provided on page 175, where you will also record your Moving
Day results 16 weeks from now. You will repeat the same testing protocol on Moving Day at the end of Phase 4. The only
difference is that your results will be much better!

I recommend that you do your pretesting on a Saturday.
This will allow you to have a day of rest before you start
Phase 1 on Monday. This chapter provides all of the information you need to complete the first four weeks of the Maximum
Strength Program. All of the Phase 1 strength exercises are
explained and illustrated. A detailed schedule of strength-
training sessions, which emphasize straight sets, and energy
workout recommendations are given at the end of the chapter.

PRETESTING (AKA PACKING DAY)

Before tackling your first set of performance tests, you'll need to
get your body weight in just a pair of underwear, preferably first

thing in the morning. At this time, you'll also want to snap a few "before" pictures against which you can compare your progress four months from now, when you take your "after" photos. Once those tasks are out of the way, you can get to the fun stuff at the gym!

As you should do with any training session, begin your pretesting by getting the blood flowing with one of the mobility warm-up routines outlined in Chapter 5. Either one will do the job. After you've completed this warm-up, move on to the specific warm-ups for the tests, and the tests themselves, in the order given below. If you do your warm-up barefoot, as I recommend, don't forget to put your shoes on for the tests.

31 + 39.5
31.8 + 39.5
(39.5 + 39.5)
36.0 + 39.5
37 + 39.5

1. BROAD JUMP

The first test is the broad jump (also known as the standing long jump). To prepare for this test, extend a tape measure on the floor (fastened securely with tape) at a length of 12 to 14 feet. I don't expect you to jump 12 feet, but you don't want to feel "cramped" at all during the test. Stand normally with the toes of both feet even with the beginning of the measuring tape.

Crouch down into a partial squat, swing your arms back, and jump forward, landing on both feet. Begin with five easy jumps at 50 percent of maximal effort just to get a feel for the movement and to get the blood flowing. Once you're feeling looser, go ahead and take a jump at 85 to 90 percent of your best effort, just to get a number on the board. Measure your jumps from the (back) of the heel of the leg that is furthest back upon landing (ideally, your two feet will land evenly). Mark off your jump with a piece of tape on the floor, and then head back to the starting line. Take three more attempts at 100 percent maximal effort, recording your best jump of the day as your official distance.

Standing Long Jump
5 @ 50%
1 @ 85–90%
3 @ 100%

2. BOX SQUAT

→ Wide stance really bugs my adductors — focus on widening the stance + loosening em before Moving Day.

For the box squat (described and illustrated on page 81–82), you'll warm up by doing a set of eight reps with just the bar, and then you'll add a small number of plates and do five more easy reps after a break of one minute. Next, perform three moderately challenging reps with a weight you could lift six or seven times before failing.

Now do three or four one-rep sets with three-minute rest periods between sets, finishing with the maximum weight you are currently capable of lifting. Do your first one-rep

TARGET
Box Squat
8 @ 45 lbs ✓
5 @ 135 lbs ✓
3 @ 225 lbs ✓
1 @ 275 lbs ✓
1 @ 285 lbs
1 @ 295 lbs ✗✓
~~1 @ 305 lbs~~ Too Risky
(etc)

ON MOVING DAY, I'LL BE BIGGER THAN MIKEY WHITING.

set with a weight that you are very confident of being able to lift once but might not be able to lift twice. Add 5 to 10 pounds to each subsequent lift until you reach your true maximum. For example, if your current box squat max is 150 pounds, your warm-up and performance test sequence might look like this:

1. Bar (45 pounds) x 8
2. 95 (bar + 25 pounds per side) x 5
3. 125 x 3 (moderately challenging)
4. 135 x 1
5. 145 x 1
6. 150 x 1 (very challenging; it'll count as your one-rep max)

Err on the side of caution and never rush through your attempts. Remember never to attempt a rep that you cannot complete with perfect form. We aren't looking for "ugly" reps. Record your results.

3. BENCH PRESS

Follow the same warm-up and performance test protocol for the bench press that you followed for the box squat. Start by lifting only the bar eight times. Next, perform three moderately challenging reps with a weight you could lift six or seven times before failing. Now do three or four one-rep sets with three-minute rest periods between sets, finishing with the maximum weight you are currently capable of lifting. Do your first one-rep set with a weight that you are very confident of being able to lift once but might not be able to lift twice. Add 5 to 10 pounds to each subsequent lift until you reach your true maximum. Record your results. See page 90–91 for a description and illustrations of proper bench press technique.

[handwritten margin notes:]
TARGET
Bench Press
8 @ 45 lbs ✓
5 @ 135 lbs ✓
3 @ 185 lbs ✓
1 @ 205 lbs
1 @ 215 lbs
1 @ 225 lbs ✓
1 @ 235 lbs ✓

4. DEADLIFT

I will preface this test with the following disclaimer: If there is one test you should consider omitting from your repertoire, the deadlift is it. The reason is that at the beginning of a resistance-training program, many people lack the flexibility needed to deadlift from the floor safely. Combine this problem with the fact that you'll be a bit fatigued from the other tests by the time that you get to the deadlift, and you have a higher potential for injury. This is one reason we'll be doing "speed deadlifts" with a lower percentage of your one-rep maximum deadlift early in this program; they give you a chance to practice the movement.

If you are *not* familiar with the lift already, do not do it. You'll still have several measures from which to gauge your progress, and you'll be able to improve your flexibility to the point where you can do the lift safely by the time this program is complete. If you *are* familiar with the lift, proceed in accordance with the guidelines below—but "call it" if your form starts to break down.

Follow the same warm-up and performance test protocol for the deadlift that you followed for the box squat and bench press, but adjust the weight for the current movement. (You will probably be able to deadlift more weight than you could box-squat or bench-press.) Start by lifting only the bar eight times to get your groove, then do two more warm-up sets of three reps with increasing weight, and then do three or four one-rep lifts with increasing weight until you hit your limit. Proper technique for the deadlift is described and illustrated on page 83–84.

5. THREE-REP MAX CHIN-UP

Proper technique for the three-rep max chin-up is described and illustrated on page 104. Warm up for this performance test by doing three body weight chin-ups. Move into the performance test by adding external resistance (in the form of weight plates attached to a weightlifting belt by a chain) and complete another set of three reps. Continue adding external resistance and doing three-rep sets until you find your maximum.

PHASE 1 STRENGTH EXERCISES

You will do 20 different strength exercises during Phase 1. The amount of resistance/weight you use in each exercise depends on how many repetitions per set are prescribed in a given session. As a general rule, use the highest level of resistance/weight you can lift for the prescribed number of repetitions with perfect form. This rule does not apply to exercises (such as scapular push-ups) that use only body weight for resistance. You will find specific training guidelines in the Phase 1 Training Schedule at the end of this chapter.

TARGET
Deadlift
8 @ 135 lbs
3 @ 225 lbs
3 @ 225 lbs
1 @ 275 lbs
~~1 @ 295 lbs~~
1 @ 335 lbs
1 @ 365 lbs
1 @ 385 lbs
TARGET
Chin-Up
(Neutral Grip)
3 @ BWt
3 @ 45
3 @ 60

Box Squat

BENEFITS: This exercise strengthens the glutes, hamstrings, quadriceps, and various core stabilizers.

SETUP: Position a box behind you in a power or squat rack. Set up under the barbell as you would for a normal squat, but allow the bar to sit a bit lower on your upper back. Pull the bar down into your traps (i.e., your upper back muscles) by tightening your lats (i.e., your large mid-back muscles) and pulling the elbows forward. Brace your core tightly and take a good gasp of air into your lungs.

ACTION: With a slightly wider stance than you'd normally use, and with your weight on the heels and outsides of your feet, sit back and not down to the box behind you, forcing the knees out to the sides as if you were squatting between your legs instead of over them. When you lower yourself correctly, you'll feel a stretch in the inner thighs and hamstrings. The box height should put you at a point where the crease of your hips is just below the kneecap in the bottom position.

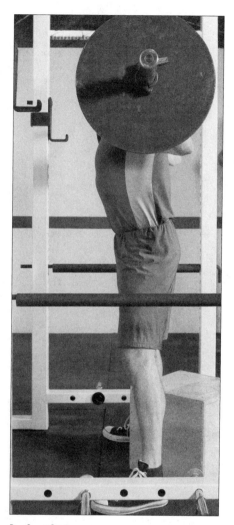

Box Squat Start

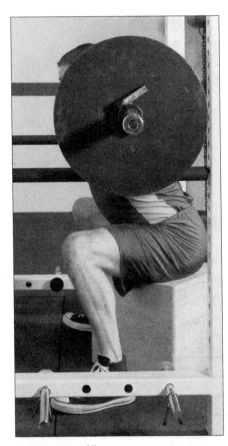

Box Squat Start Middle

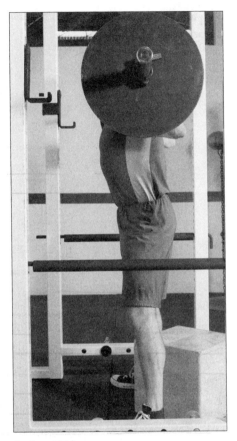

Box Squat Finish

Do not bounce off the box. Sit lightly down on it and pause without rocking backward. There will be a little forward lean in your torso in the bottom position. To stand up, continue to push through the heels, and <u>explode off the box, thinking</u> <u>about thrusting your hips forward instead</u> <u>of just extending your knees.</u> Your quads really just come along for the ride as the <u>hamstrings and glutes do the brunt of the</u> <u>work. Stand tall at the completion of each</u> <u>rep</u> before descending for your next rep.

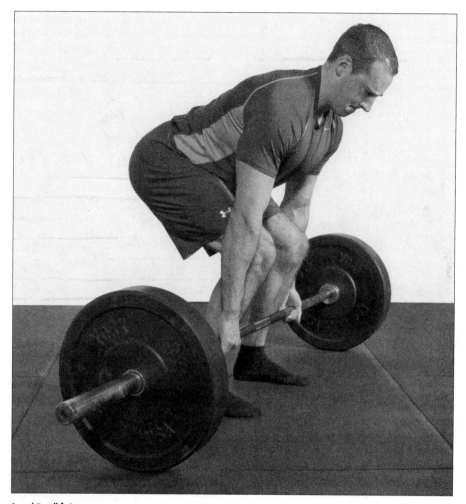

Speed Deadlift Start

Speed Deadlift

BENEFITS: This exercise strengthens the glutes, hamstrings, upper back, grip, and various core stabilizers.

SETUP: Stand facing a weighted barbell with your feet at shoulder width and your shins almost touching the bar. Squat down and, using an overhand grip, grasp the bar with the arms fully extended and close to the sides of the thighs. Think about getting your chest as high and as far forward as possible—you might have to sink your butt down a little more than you otherwise would.

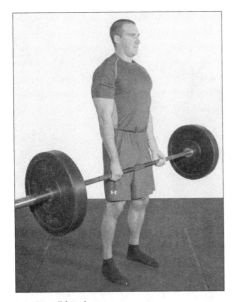

Speed Deadlift Lockout

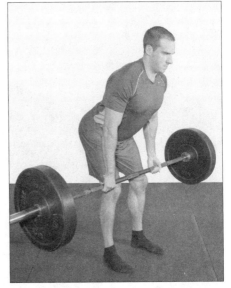

Speed Deadlift Lowering

ACTION: Drive the heels into the floor and push your hips forward as your knees extend; <u>think of pinching something between your butt cheeks at the top to lock the weight out.</u> Do not just lean back.

You initiate the lowering portion by pushing the butt back (to prestretch the hamstrings); don't worry about bending the knees until the bar has passed them. Once the bar has passed them, you can bend the knees to get the rest of the way to the floor.

The single most important component of the deadlift is maintaining a neutral spine position. You should not round over at any point. If you don't have the flexibility to pull from the floor without rounding yet, elevate the plates a bit (with an aerobics step, or by stacking them on some other plates).

<u>Once the weight gets challenging,</u> you'll notice that your grip will start to become an issue. <u>I recommend getting some chalk for your hands, and also trying out the alternate grip</u> (overhand with one hand, underhand with the other). In certain deadlift variations, you'll want to use straps, but <u>you should never rely on them when performing conventional deadlifts from the floor.</u> (STRAPS) Here, in Phase 1, you'll be performing what we call <u>speed deadlifts.</u> The idea is to <u>use a lighter load (50 to 65 percent of your one-rep max)</u> in order to develop technique and faster bar speed on the lift.

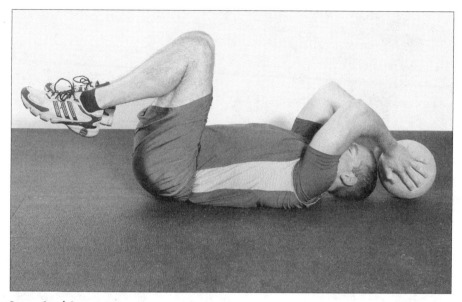

Reverse Crunch Start

Reverse Crunch

BENEFITS: This exercise targets the external obliques, commonly referred to as the lower abs, and helps to correct forward pelvic tilt—a common postural imbalance.

SETUP: Lie face up on the floor with your knees sharply bent, your feet elevated a couple of inches off the floor, and your arms extended straight overhead.

ACTION: Contract your abs and attempt to pull the knees toward the elbows without allowing the ankles to lose contact with your butt. The only motion should be a posterior tilt of the pelvis; you'll feel it in your lower abs. Your arms shouldn't move. At first, almost everyone does this exercise incorrectly by letting the legs

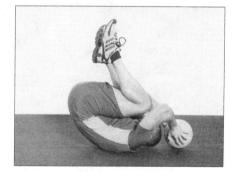

Reverse Crunch Finish

drop too far and just using the hip flexors. To avoid cheating when you're initially learning this exercise, hold onto something (e.g., a medicine ball or dumbbell) behind your head to keep yourself in place. As you get more proficient with the movement, you can go to a lighter implement or just leave it out altogether.

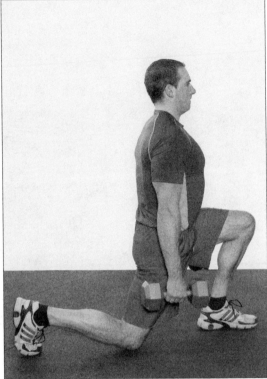

Walking Dumbbell Lunge Step 1

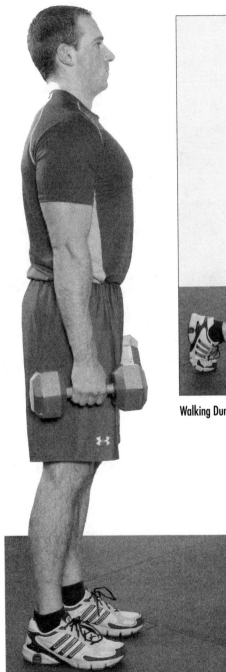

Walking Dumbbell Lunge Start

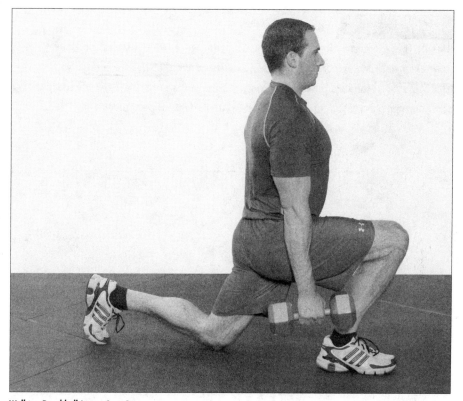

Walking Dumbbell Lunge Step 2

Walking Dumbbell Lunge

BENEFITS: This exercise strengthens the glutes, hamstrings, quadriceps, grip, and various core stabilizers.

SETUP: Stand normally holding dumbbells at your sides.

ACTION: Take a long stride forward, landing on your heel and decelerating with the strength of your glutes, hamstrings, and quads. Sink into the lunge until the knee of your trailing leg lightly grazes the floor, and then push through the front foot's heel to propel yourself forward into the next step. Be sure to keep the chest up and shoulder blades pulled back throughout this movement.

Prone Bridge

BENEFITS: This exercise helps to build muscular endurance in key core stabilizers.

SETUP: Assume a standard push-up position with your upper body weight supported on your forearms instead of your palms. Maintain a 90-degree bend in your elbows and make sure they are placed directly underneath the shoulders.

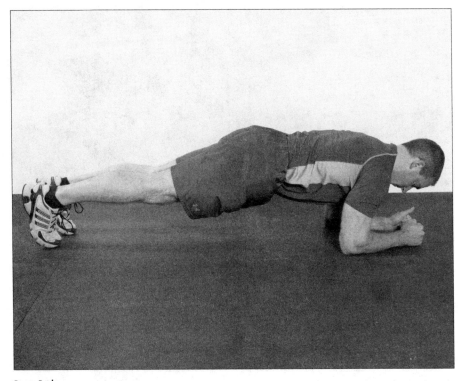

Prone Bridge

ACTION: Brace your entire core area and keep your hips up and in line with your legs and torso. Think "forearms and toes" with the hips held firm. Hold this position for the amount of time designated in the Phase 1 Strength-Training Schedule (see page 108). If the two-legged version feels too easy and you're meeting your time goal without a problem, switch to a version where one foot is raised slightly off the floor.

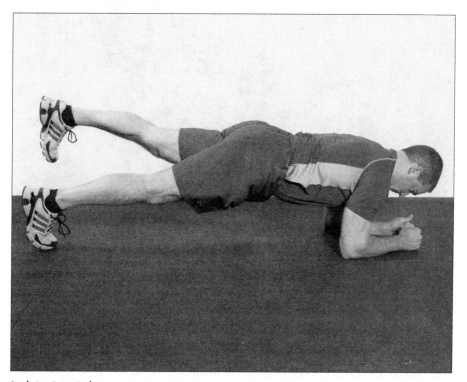

Single-Leg Prone Bridge

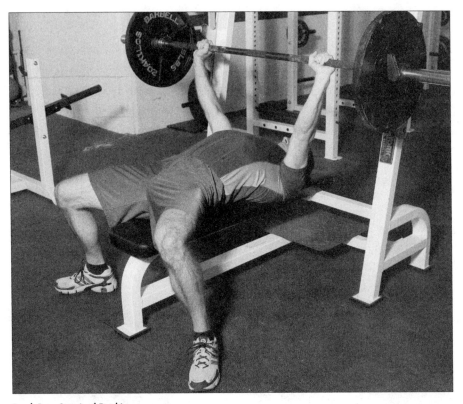

Bench Press Start (and Finish)

Bench Press

BENEFITS: This exercise primarily strengthens the chest, shoulders, and triceps, although there is considerable involvement of the upper back, lower body, and core musculature when the exercise is performed correctly.

SETUP: Line up on the bench so that the very top of your head is directly underneath the bar. Retract your shoulder blades hard. Now slide your body toward the head end of the bench until your eyes are directly under the bar. Keep your shoulder blades pulled down and back. Your rib cage should pop right up. Set your feet underneath your knees, not out in front. This position will put your back in its natural arch.

ACTION: Grasp the bar with your hands placed roughly 1.5 times your shoulder width apart, and get a good handoff

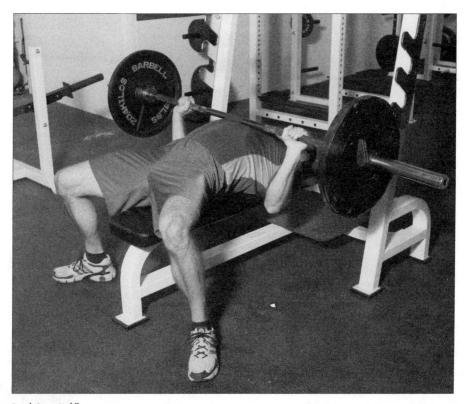

Bench Press Middle

from someone so that you don't lose the tight upper back you've established. Keep those shoulder blades back and down!

As you lower the bar, keep the upper arms at a 45-degree angle to the torso, and tuck the elbows instead of letting them flare out, as it's easier on the shoulders. Get a big gulp of air so that the belly and chest rise up to meet the bar as it descends. Lower the bar until it lightly touches your chest.

As you press the bar up (driving through your heels as well), imagine trying to push yourself away from it (through the bench). You can also think of spreading the bar to activate the triceps a bit more. As you lock the weight out, do not excessively protract the shoulder blades; you shouldn't lose your tightness in that area prior to descending into the next rep.

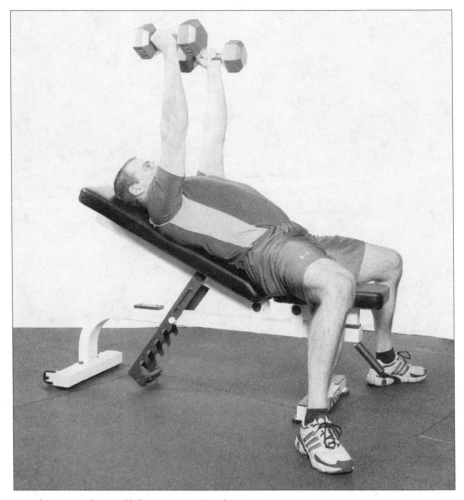

Neutral-Grip Low-Incline Dumbbell Press Start (and Finish)

Neutral-Grip Low-Incline Dumbbell Press

BENEFITS: This exercise primarily strengthens the chest, shoulders, and triceps.

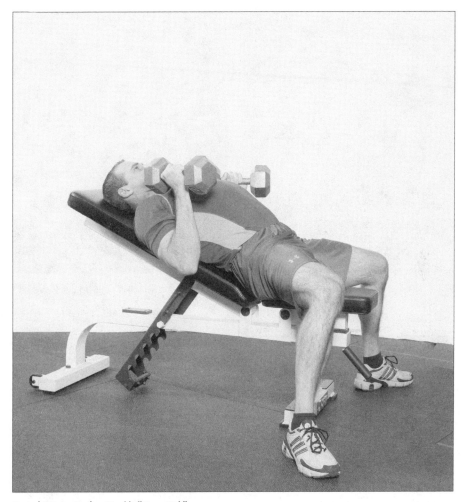

Neutral-Grip Low-Incline Dumbbell Press Middle

SETUP: Set your incline bench at a <u>30- to 45-degree angle.</u> Sit on the bench with your back and head resting against the incline. Begin with your arms extended straight toward the ceiling, a dumbbell in each hand, and your <u>palms facing each other.</u>

ACTION: <u>Lower the dumbbells until they are just above and outside your shoulders. Now press the dumbbells straight up— not forward—to lock out, being careful not to let the shoulder blades loosen up.</u> Stay tight just as you did on the regular bench press.

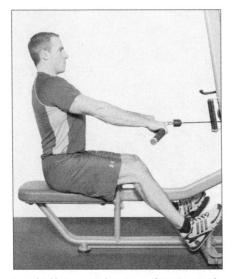

Seated Cable Row—Medium Pronated Grip Start (and Finish)

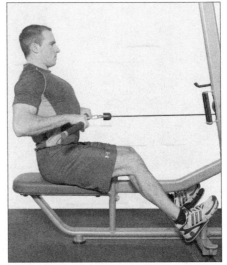

Seated Cable Row—Medium Pronated Grip Middle

Seated Cable Row: Medium Pronated Grip

BENEFITS: This exercise strengthens several upper back muscles—the lats, upper/middle/lower trapezius, and rhomboids—as well as the elbow flexors (most notably, the biceps) and grip.

SETUP: Sit at a cable row station with a slight bend in the knees. Grab the handle with both hands, using a shoulder-width, overhand grip. Keep the chest out, shoulders back, and eyes straight ahead so that you're sitting up tall.

ACTION: Think "shoulder blades back and down" as you pull the handle to your stomach. Extend your arms to return to the starting position.

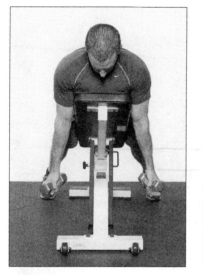

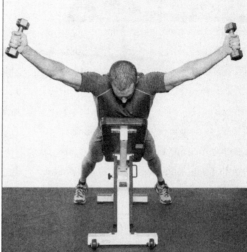

Prone Trap Raise Start **Prone Trap Raise Finish**

Prone Trap Raise

BENEFITS: This exercise strengthens the lower trapezius, which is crucial for ideal upward rotation of the shoulder blades during overhead movements.

SETUP: Lie face down on a 45-degree incline bench with a light dumbbell in each hand and your arms hanging toward the floor. Imagine your head is in the 12 o'clock position on a clock face.

ACTION: Keeping the thumbs up, raise the arms to 10 o'clock and 2 o'clock without bending the elbows. You should feel the effort predominantly in the mid-back area. If you find yourself "cramping" up in the upper traps and neck, you're shrugging too much. If that's the case, drop the weight and just focus on getting a feel for the movement with the weight of your arms only.

Side-Lying External Rotation

BENEFITS: This exercise strengthens the infraspinatus, teres minor, and posterior deltoid—three muscles that must be strong for the shoulder to functional effectively.

SETUP: Lie on your side on the floor or on a bench with your bottom arm extending in front of you. Begin with the upper part of your top arm resting snuggly against your side, the elbow bent 90 degrees, and a lightweight plate or dumbbell in the top-side hand.

ACTION: Rotate the shoulder of your top-side arm and swing the weight upward as far as you can comfortably go. Keep the elbow locked against your side. You'll feel the effort in the back of your shoulder. Return to the starting position.

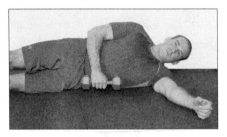

Side-Lying External Rotation Start

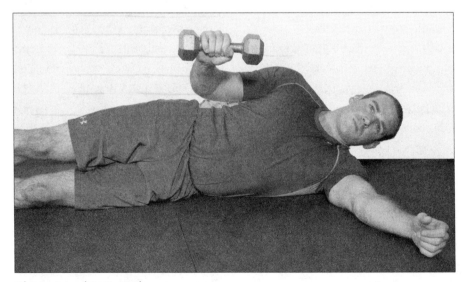

Side-Lying External Rotation Finish

Side Bridge

BENEFITS: This exercise builds endurance in key core stabilizers, most notably the internal and external obliques.

SETUP: Lie on your side on the floor with the elbow of your bottom arm bent 90 degrees and only the forearm in contact with the floor, so that your torso is propped up. Your legs are straight and your feet stacked.

ACTION: Brace the core tightly and lift your hips until your body forms a straight line from head to toe. Don't let the hips sag. Hold this position for the designated amount of time.

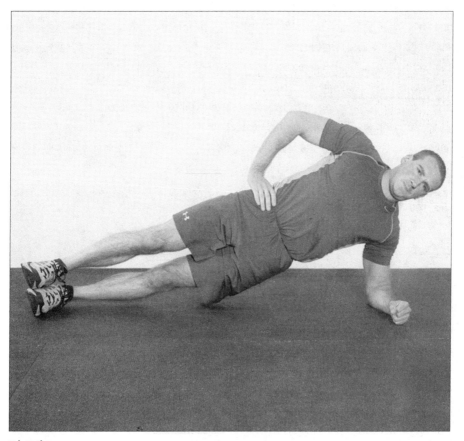

Side Bridge

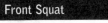

Front Squat

BENEFITS: This exercise strengthens the quadriceps, glutes, hamstrings, and several core stabilizers.

SETUP: Cross your arms at the wrists, and then take your thumbs to the edge of the knurl in the center of the bar, which will be set up in a power/squat rack at shoulder height. From there, dip down under the bar and force your elbows high so the bar sits in the "divot" you've created in your shoulders by elevating the elbows. If you have the bar in the right spot, it'll be just short of choking you. Don't worry, the discomfort will go away after a few weeks as you get used to it. I should note that some lifters do prefer the clean grip over the cross-face grip, and below, I've included photos of both so that you can experiment and choose which of the two feels best for you. In both cases, the bar is "racked" on the entire shoulder girdle, not simply supported by the arms.

ACTION: Take a big gulp of air into your lungs, tighten your core, and lift the bar off the rack by standing up fully. Take a step backward and set your feet slightly farther than shoulder-width apart and turn your toes out slightly, if that's more comfortable for you. Break at the hips and knees simultaneously to squat down as deeply as you can without rounding over along the spine. Keep the weight on the mid-foot, not the toes. Without bouncing in the bottom position, reverse your direction by using the strength of your quads, glutes, and hamstrings to accelerate the bar all the way up to lockout.

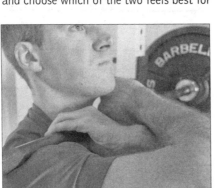

Cross-Face Grip

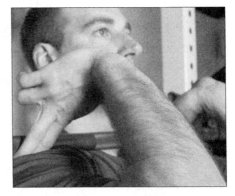

Clean Grip

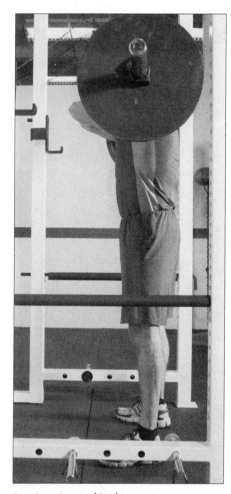

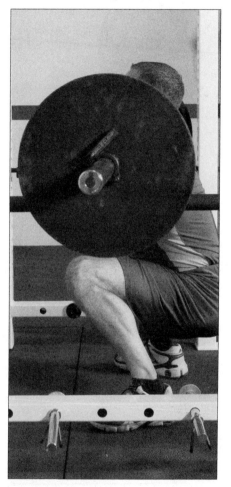

Front Squat Start (and Finish)

Front Squat Middle

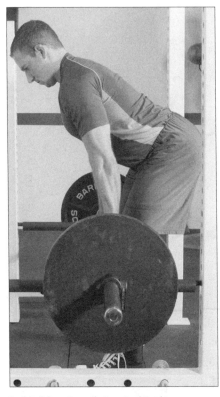

Rack Pull from Kneecaps Start (and Finish)

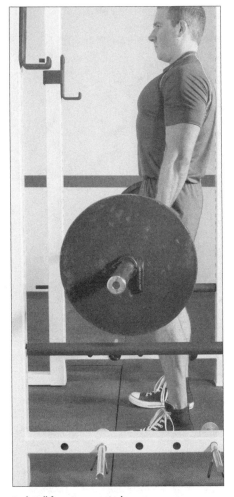

Rack Pull from Kneecaps

BENEFITS: This exercise strengthens the glutes, hamstrings, upper back, grip, and various core stabilizers. It's an excellent movement for those who aren't flexible enough to deadlift from the floor.

SETUP: This is just a partial deadlift from the pins in the power rack.

ACTION: Perform a deadlift exactly as

Rack Pull from Kneecaps Lockout

described on page 83–84, except with the bar set at knee height. Reset the bar on the pins after each rep. Note that you'll be able to use more weight than with conventional deadlifts from the floor.

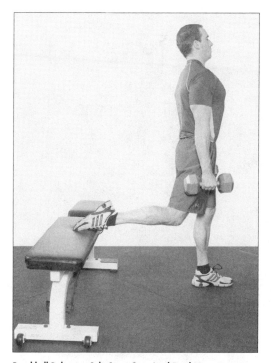

Dumbbell Bulgarian Split Squat Start (and Finish)

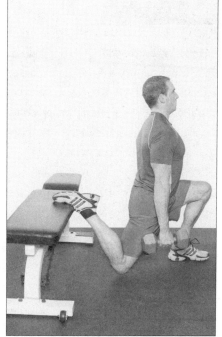

Dumbbell Bulgarian Split Squat Middle

Dumbbell Bulgarian Split Squat

BENEFITS: This exercise strengthens the glutes, hamstrings, quadriceps, grip, and various core stabilizers.

SETUP: Position a bench roughly three feet behind you. Stand normally with your arms hanging at your sides and a dumbbell in each hand. Reach backward with one leg and place the top of that foot on the bench.

ACTION: Break at the knee of the forward leg and lower yourself down into a split-squat position. In the bottom position, the knee of your trailing leg should be just short of touching the floor, with the torso upright and shoulders pulled back. You'll feel a great stretch on the front of the hip and thigh of the trailing leg. Your weight should be almost completely on the mid-foot of the forward leg with the toe of the back foot just helping you to maintain balance. Push through the front leg to return to the starting position, where you'll stand upright by fully extending the hip and knee. After completing a full set, reverse your position and work the opposite leg.

Pull-Through

BENEFITS: The pull-through is a great exercise for targeting the posterior chain—hamstrings, glutes, and hip adductors—without placing a ton of stress on the back. It's also excellent for teaching appropriate lower-back and hip movement for exercises such as deadlifts and box squats.

SETUP: Stand facing away from a cable column with the rope attachment set in the bottom position. Set your feet slightly farther than shoulder-width apart so that you have room to reach between your legs with both arms fully extended, and grasp the rope. Bend your knees slightly and bend forward slightly at the hips to counterbalance the pull of the rope. Be sure to keep your weight on your heels.

ACTION: To initiate the movement, let the weight pull your hips back as if someone had a rope tied around your waist and was pulling you backward. Now begin tilting your torso forward from the hips (not the waist) and allow the weight to pull your extended arms between your legs. Avoid rounding your back. The lowering phase ends when the torso is just short of parallel with the floor, at which point you'll push through the heels and use your posterior chain to pull the rope forward between your legs and straighten your body back to the starting position. Push your hips forward and squeeze your glutes to lock out. Stand upright; don't lean back!

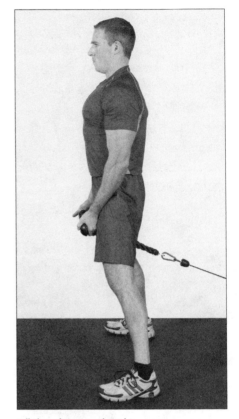

Pull-Through Start (and Finish)

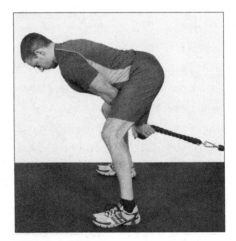

Pull-Through Middle

One-Arm Dumbbell Push Press

BENEFITS: This exercise strengthens the shoulders, triceps, and several core stabilizers.

SETUP: Stand normally with a dumbbell in one hand and your arm folded so that the weight is just above your shoulder.

ACTION: Sink into a quarter-squat position and then extend your legs powerfully to give the dumbbell upward momentum. The moment your knees lock out, forcefully contract your shoulder and press the dumbbell overhead. Lower the dumbbell back to your shoulder. Complete the designated number of repetitions, and then repeat the exercise with the other arm.

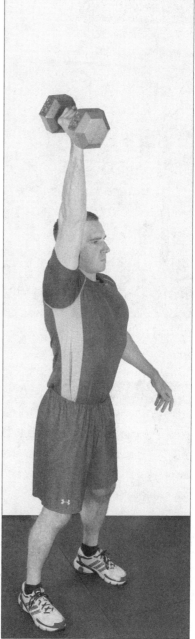

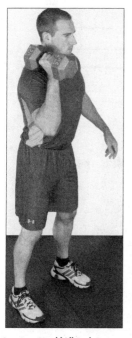

One-Arm Dumbbell Push Press Start

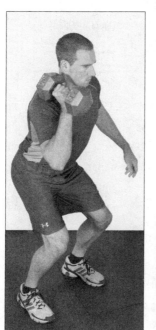

One-Arm Dumbbell Push Press Middle

One-Arm Dumbbell Push Press Finish

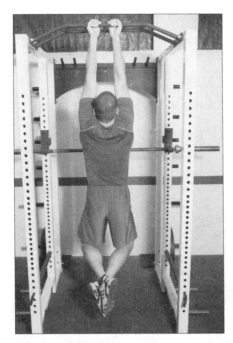

Close-Grip Chin-Up Start

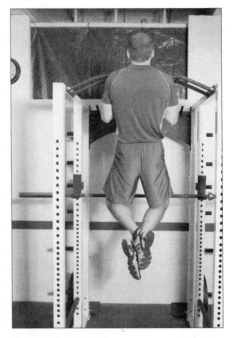

Close-Grip Chin-Up Finish

Close-Grip Chin-Up

BENEFIT: This exercise strengthens the lats, biceps, and grip, plus several core stabilizers.

SETUP: Position your hands roughly six inches apart on a chin-up bar with the palms facing you.

ACTION: Pull your body upward until your chin clears the bar, and then lower yourself back to the starting position. To add weight, wear a weight vest or use a chain and/or dipping belt to hang a dumbbell or weight plate from your waist.

Push-Up

BENEFITS: The push-up may seem rudimentary in the context of this program, but the sad truth is that 95 percent of gym goers have no idea how to perform the movement correctly. The beauty of this movement is that it not only requires minimal equipment but also allows you to train the muscles of the upper body in closed-chain motion (hands fixed, body moving) instead of the more traditional open chain (body fixed, arms moving, e.g., the bench press). The push-up strengthens the chest, shoulders, and triceps.

SETUP: Everyone knows the push-up starting position, but most people take their hands out too wide. Position the hands just outside shoulder width. Imagine your body being a straight line from ankles to neck; don't allow the hips to sag or the butt to stick up too high. The chin should be tucked (double chin) so that your head is close to being in line with your body.

ACTION: Lower your chest to within an inch of the floor. As you do, think about pulling your chest (not your hips or chin) down to the floor. If you do the exercise right, you'll actually feel the muscles in your upper back working to pull you down into this position. The elbows should be set at a 45-degree angle to the body; this position is much easier on the shoulders. Look straight at the floor the entire time, and keep the core braced tightly (as though someone is about to punch you in the stomach, and you're trying to protect yourself). Press back to the starting position.

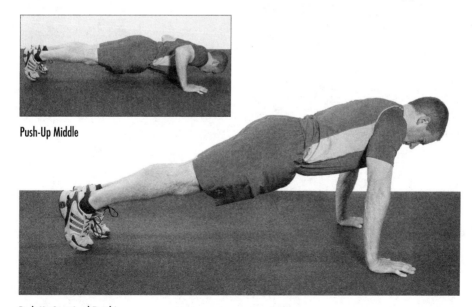

Push-Up Middle

Push-Up Start (and Finish)

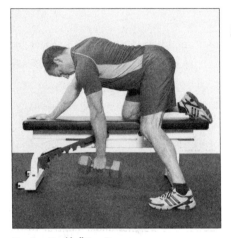

One-Arm Dumbbell Row Start

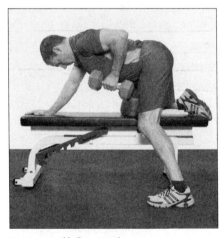

One-Arm Dumbbell Row Finish

One-Arm Dumbbell Row

BENEFITS: This exercise strengthens several upper-back muscles—the lats, upper/middle/lower trapezius, and rhomboids—as well as the elbow flexors (most notably, the biceps) and grip.

SETUP: Place your left hand and left knee on a bench so that your torso is parallel to the ground with the spine in a neutral position (not rounded). Position your right foot on the floor next to the bench. Grasp a dumbbell in your right hand and begin with your right arm extended straight toward the floor.

ACTION: Retract your shoulder blade and bend your elbow to raise the dumbbell up to your side. Be sure to keep the elbow close to the body, and avoid jerking the weight or rotating the torso to create upward momentum. Lower the weight back to the starting position. After completing the designated number of repetitions, reverse your position and work the other side.

Kneeling Cable External Rotation

BENEFITS: This exercise strengthens the infraspinatus, teres minor, and posterior deltoid—three muscles that are crucial to overall shoulder health.

SETUP: Kneel on both knees while facing a double-sided cable column (two weight stacks) with the D-handles positioned down near the floor. Grasp one handle in each hand with your upper arms positioned straight out to the sides, parallel to the floor, and the elbows flexed 90 degrees so that your forearms are pointing toward the weight stacks. The weight plates should be elevated in this starting position so that there's tension on the cables.

ACTION: Externally rotate the shoulders and swing your forearms 90 degrees upward, so that they are now pointing toward the ceiling (scarecrow position). Keep your chest high and your upper arms locked in position throughout this movement. Lower the weights under control to the starting position, and repeat for reps.

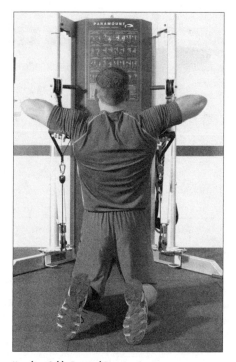

Kneeling Cable External Rotation Start

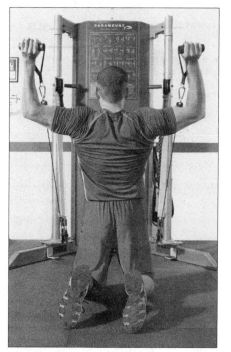

Kneeling Cable External Rotation Finish

PHASE 1 TRAINING SCHEDULE

	WEEK 1 HIGH	WEEK 2 MEDIUM	WEEK 3 VERY HIGH	WEEK 4 LOW
SUNDAY: REST OR ENERGY WORKOUT				
MONDAY: LOWER BODY				
A Box Squat	5x4	4x4	8x3	3x3
B Speed Deadlift	8x2 @50% 1RM	8x2 @55% 1RM	10x2 @60% 1RM	3x2 @65% 1RM
C Walking Dumbbell Lunge	4x8 /side	3x8 /side	4x8 /side	2x8 /side (easy)
D1 Reverse Crunch	3x12	3x12	3x12	3x12
D2 Prone Bridge	3x30s	3x30s	3x30s	3x30s
TUESDAY: REST OR ENERGY WORKOUT				
WEDNESDAY: UPPER BODY				
A Bench Press	5x4	4x4	8x3	3x3
B1 Neutral-Grip Low-Incline DB Press	3x10	3x9	3x10	2x10
B2 Seated Cable Row: Medium Pronated Grip	4x10	4x9	4x10	3x10
C1 Prone Trap Raise	3x12	3x12	3x12	3x12
C2 Side-Lying External Rotation	3x12 /side	3x12 /side	3x12 /side	3x12 /side
D Side Bridge	3x30s /side	3x30s /side	3x30s /side	3x30s /side

	WEEK 1 HIGH	WEEK 2 MEDIUM	WEEK 3 VERY HIGH	WEEK 4 LOW
THURSDAY: REST OR ENERGY WORKOUT				
FRIDAY: LOWER BODY				
A Front Squat	4x6	4x6	6x6	3x6
B Rack Pull from Kneecaps	4x6	3x6	4x6	2x6
C DB Bulgarian Split Squat	3x6 /side	3x5 /side	4x6 /side	2x6 /side
D1 Pull-Through	3x10	3x10	3x10	2x10
D2 Reverse Crunch	3x12	3x12	3x12	3x12
SATURDAY: UPPER BODY				
A1 One-Arm DB Push Press	4x6 /side	4x6 /side	6x6 /side	3x6 /side
A2 Close-Grip Chin-Up	4x6	3x6	4x6	3x6
B1 Push-Up	3x10	3x12	4x10	3x8
B2 One-Arm DB Row	3x8	3x7	4x8	3x7
C1 Kneeling Cable External Rotation	3x12	3x12	3x12	3x12
C2 Side Bridge	3x30s /side	3x30s /side	3x30s /side	3x30s /side

Key to Notations: 5x4 = Five sets of four repetitions, and so forth.
3x30s = Three sets of 30 seconds.

PHASE 1 STRENGTH-TRAINING SCHEDULE

Here is your four-week strength-training schedule for Phase 1. Remember to begin each session by doing one of the two warm-ups presented in Chapter 5. In each exercise involving external weight/resistance, use the highest level of weight/resistance you can lift for the designated number of repetitions with perfect form. In exercises involving no external resistance (reverse crunch, etc.), simply perform the designated number of repetitions. Between sets, rest as long as necessary to perform the next set at the same level of performance, but not longer. When you see "A1" and "A2" or "B1" and "B2," etc., you should alternate between those two exercises.

PHASE 1 ENERGY
WORKOUT RECOMMENDATIONS

Following are energy workout recommendations for Phase 1. Separate recommendations are provided for each of the three somatotypes discussed in Chapter 3.

Ectomorphs

TUESDAY AND THURSDAY. Technique practice of your choice (see page 24 for a sample technique practice session) with 30 percent of one-rep max, then 20 minutes of low-intensity cardio (stationary cycling, running, etc., at 60 to 70 percent of max heart rate).

Mesomorphs

IMMEDIATELY FOLLOWING EACH STRENGTH-TRAINING SESSION. Ten minutes of low-intensity cardio (stationary cycling, running, etc., at 60 to 70 percent of max heart rate).

TUESDAY. Fifteen minutes (excluding warm-up and cooldown) of high-intensity intervals on a 15-seconds work/45-seconds rest cycle on the elliptical trainer, bicycle, or rower. Running is your best choice, if you can manage it.

THURSDAY. Technique practice (see page 24 for a sample technique practice session) with 30 percent of one-rep max, then 20 minutes low-intensity cardio (stationary cycling, running, etc., at 60 to 70 percent of max heart rate).

Endomorphs

IMMEDIATELY FOLLOWING EACH STRENGTH-TRAINING SESSION. Ten minutes of low-intensity cardio (stationary cycling, running, etc., at 60 to 70 percent of max heart rate).

SATURDAY. Replace low-intensity posttraining cardio with 10 minutes of high-intensity intervals on a 20-seconds work/40-seconds rest cycle on the elliptical trainer, bicycle, rower, or on foot (running).

TUESDAY. Fifteen minutes (excluding warm-up and cooldown) of high-intensity intervals on a 15-seconds work/45-seconds rest cycle on the elliptical trainer, bicycle, rower, or on foot (running).

THURSDAY. Technique practice of your choice (see page 24 for a sample technique practice session) with 30 percent of one-rep max, then 20 minutes of low-intensity cardio (stationary cycling, running, etc., at 60 to 70 percent of max heart rate).

CHAPTER 7

PHASE 2: BUILD

I f you thought Phase 1 was challenging, brace yourself for Phase 2. And if you thought the first four weeks of the Maximum Strength Program were fun, get ready to have a blast during the next four weeks. This chapter provides all of the information you need to build on the foundation you laid down in Phase 1. You will experience further increases in mobility, muscle balance, muscle size, and strength performance.

All of the strength exercises are described and illustrated, and a detailed schedule of training sessions, which emphasize cluster training and energy workout recommendations, are given at the end of the chapter.

PHASE 2 STRENGTH EXERCISES

Like Phase 1, this phase includes 20 different strength exercises, with minimal overlap with Phase 1. The amount of resistance/weight you use in each exercise depends on how many repetitions per set are prescribed in a given session. As a general rule, use the highest level of resistance/weight with which you can complete the prescribed number of repetitions with perfect form. This rule does not apply to exercises that use only body weight for resistance, such as the reverse crunch. You will find specific training guidelines in the Phase 2 Strength-Training Schedule at the end of the chapter.

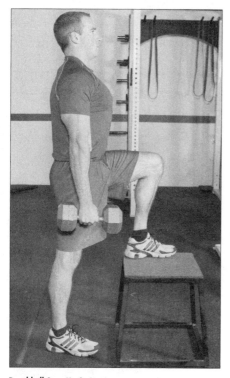

Dumbbell Step-Up Start

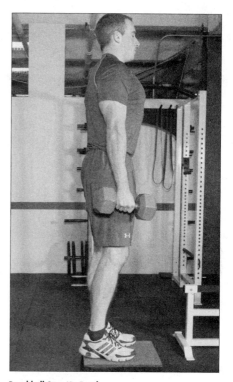

Dumbbell Step-Up Finish

Front Squat

See Phase 1, page 98.

Dumbbell Step-Up

BENEFITS: This exercise strengthens the glutes, hamstrings, quadriceps, grip, and various core stabilizers.

SETUP: Stand facing a box with one foot on top of it and one foot on the floor. The box should have a height that puts the crease of the hip of your stepping leg just below the level of your knee. Hold a dumbbell in each hand with your arms extended at your sides.

ACTION: Push through the heel of your stepping leg and use your glutes and hamstrings to straighten the leg and pull your body upward. Briefly place the foot of the nonworking leg next to the foot of the stepping leg on the box. Step back with the nonworking leg, controlling your descent with the strength of the working leg. Keep the foot of the working leg on the box for the designated number of reps, then rest before completing a set in the reverse position. In other words, don't alternate leg positions between reps.

Bar Rollout

BENEFITS: This exercise strengthens several key core stabilizers, most notably the rectus abdominus and lats.

SETUP: Place a weighted barbell on the floor. Kneel down in front of it with your hands just outside shoulder width and an overhand grip on the bar.

ACTION: Make the abs as rigid as possible and push the bar so that it rolls forward away from you. Go out to the point where your lower back wants to sag, but before it can, squeeze the abs to return to the starting position. You'll also feel the effort in your lats. Think of this exercise as a pure stabilization movement where only the arms are moving.

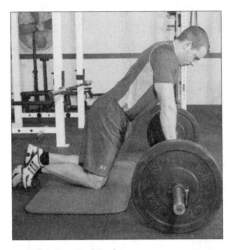

Bar Rollout Start (and Finish)

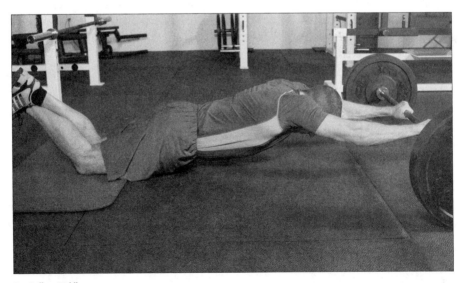

Bar Rollout Middle

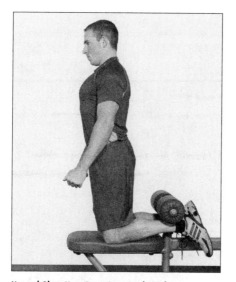

Natural Glute-Ham Raise Start (and Finish)

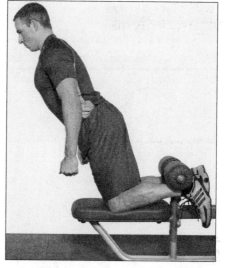

Natural Glute-Ham Raise Lowering

Natural Glute-Ham Raise

BENEFITS: This exercise strengthens the hamstrings, glutes, and gastrocnemius (one of the calf muscles).

SETUP: There are two ways to perform this exercise. Option 1: Lie face down on the floor and have a partner press your lower legs down into the floor so that your body can move only from the knee up. Option 2: Kneel on the bench of a lat pulldown or seated calf-raise machine facing the opposite direction you would normally face, and hook your feet under the pads.

ACTION: Option 1: Contract your hamstrings and lift your body (from knees to head) upward until you are in a fully upright kneeling position. Lower yourself back to the floor. Option 2: Tilt your body forward (from knees to head) until your legs are fully extended. Contract your

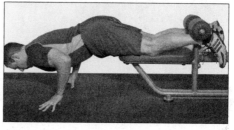

Natural Glute-Ham Raise Bottom

hamstrings and pull your body back to the starting position. For most people, a push-off with the hands to the floor in the bottom position is necessary to assist the hamstrings.

With both options, try to keep your torso erect throughout the movement, and then use the hamstrings to pull your body up and use the glutes to finish the movement (by tilting the pelvis back; just think of popping the hips forward to get your body upright).

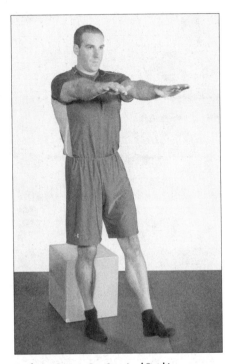

Single-Leg Squat to Box Start (and Finish)

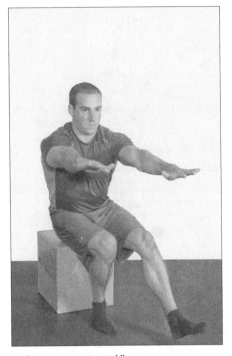

Single-Leg Squat to Box Middle

Single-Leg Squat (Pistol) to Box

BENEFITS: This exercise is a fantastic balance developer because it challenges frontal plane stability. It also strengthens the quadriceps, glutes, hamstrings, and several core stabilizers.

SETUP: Stand on one foot, approximately six inches in front of a box or bench, with both arms extended in front of you.

ACTION: With the nonworking leg held out in front of you, grip the floor with your foot as if you were trying to pick it up like a basketball, and initiate the lowering phase by pushing your hips back. Be conscious of not allowing the knee to fall inward to a knock-kneed position. Keep the chest out and shoulders back with the arms out in front. When you make contact with the bench or box with your glutes, quickly reverse your direction and return to the starting position. This contact should be a "tap and go" and not a "thud and push."

For most people, this movement will feel extremely awkward and difficult at first, so start with a higher bench or box and gradually work your way down. You might even get good enough to go all the way down without a bench or box, eventually!

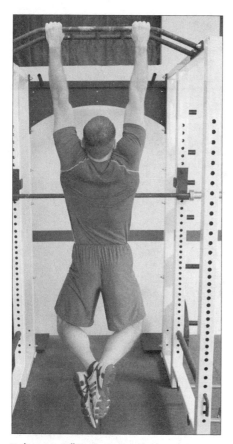

Medium Grip Pull-Up Start

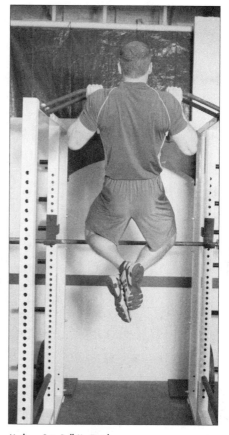

Medium Grip Pull-Up Finish

Weighted Medium-Grip Pull-Up

BENEFIT: This exercise strengthens the lats, elbow flexors (including the biceps), and grip, plus several core stabilizers.

SETUP: Set up the same way you set up for the close-grip chin-up (see Phase 1, page 104), but this time position the hands approximately shoulder-width apart on the bar and use an overhand grip. Wear a weight vest or use a chain and/or dipping belt to hang a dumbbell or weight plate from your waist. Use the maximum amount of weight with which you can complete the prescribed number of repetitions in a given set.

ACTION: Perform this exercise the same way you perform the close-grip chin-up, using the alternative grip just described.

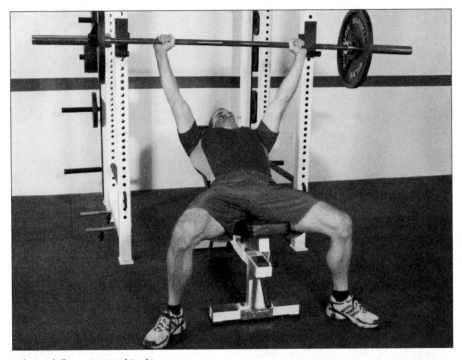

Incline Barbell Press Start (and Finish)

Incline Barbell Press

BENEFITS: This exercise strengthens primarily the chest, shoulders, and triceps.

SETUP: Set up for this exercise the same way you set up for the bench press (see Phase 1, page 90), except on an incline bench set at 30 to 45 degrees.

ACTION: Perform this exercise the same way you perform the bench press, but allow the bar to touch a little higher on the chest. As with the bench press, make sure that you have a spotter to hand the bar off to you.

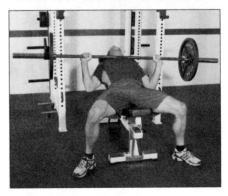

Incline Barbell Press Middle

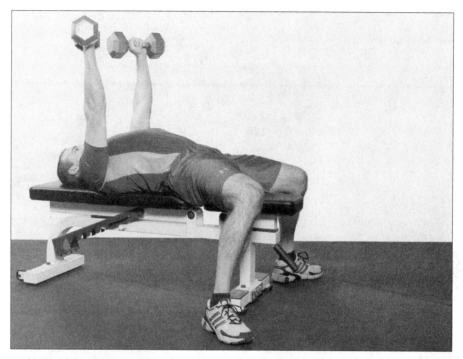

Dumbbell Bench Press Start (and Finish)

Dumbbell Bench Press

BENEFITS: This exercise strengthens primarily the chest, shoulders, and triceps.

SETUP: Lie face up on an exercise bench with your arms extended straight toward the ceiling and a dumbbell in each hand, palms facing your feet. Position your feet underneath your knees on the floor. Tighten your shoulder blades and try to keep them in contact with the bench.

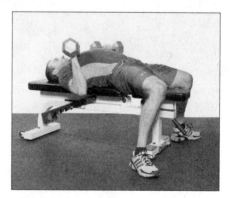

Dumbbell Bench Press Middle

ACTION: Bend your elbows and lower them toward the floor until the dumbbells are almost touching your shoulders. Keep your shoulder blades tight. Contract your chest muscles and press the dumbbells back to the starting position.

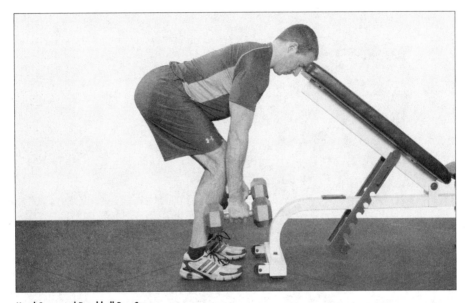

Head-Supported Dumbbell Row Start

Head-Supported Dumbbell Row

BENEFITS: This exercise strengthens several upper-back muscles—the lats, upper/middle/lower trapezius, and rhomboids—as well as the elbow flexors (most notably, the biceps) and grip.

SETUP: Set up a bench in an incline position so that the top is approximately at the height of your hips. Stand behind the head of the bench and facing it. Bend forward from the hips and rest your forehead on the top of the inclined segment of the bench. Begin with both arms extended straight toward the floor and a dumbbell in each hand.

ACTION: Contract your upper back muscles and draw the weights up to the sides of

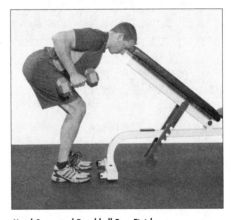

Head-Supported Dumbbell Row Finish

your rib cage. Keep the chin tucked and chest out, and make sure that the elbows remain close to the body as you pull your shoulder blades back. Lower the weights back to the starting position.

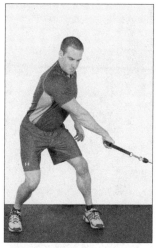 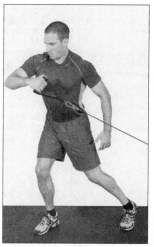

Cable Backhand Start   Cable Backhand Middle   Cable Backhand Finish

Cable Backhand

BENEFITS: This is an excellent exercise for integrating several joints in a complex, co-operative movement and a great exercise for shoulder health as well.

SETUP: To perform this movement with the right arm, stand with your left side facing a cable column and hold a D-handle in your right hand. Begin with your right arm reaching across your body with the hand roughly at the height of your left pants pocket and your hips rotated slightly in the direction of the cable column.

ACTION: Pull the handle across your body from low to high as though you're hitting a backhand tennis shot. You're combining hip rotation with core stabilization, upper-arm abduction and external rotation, scapular retraction and upward rotation, and elbow extension. Make sure you don't round over your back, and that you're rotating at the

hips and not the lower back. When this exercise is performed correctly, you'll feel it in the glutes, posterior shoulder girdle, and triceps. The palm faces down in the starting position and forward/up in the finish position. Lower the weight under control back to the starting position. After completing a full set, work the opposite side.

Broad Jump

BENEFITS: The broad jump develops explosive power throughout the lower body.

SETUP: Set up the same way you set up for your broad jump performance test during pretesting, but don't worry about the measurement part.

ACTION: Perform this exercise the same way you did during pretesting, with one twist: Instead of doing a single jump, do sets of five consecutive broad jumps with short pauses between reps.

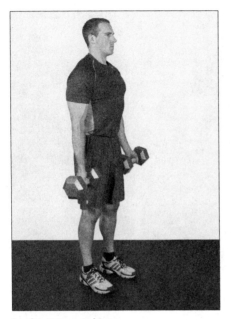

Standing Zottman Curl Start

Standing Zottman Curl Top

Standing Zottman Curl

BENEFITS: This movement strengthens all of the elbow flexors, including the biceps, brachialis, and brachioradialis, which are crucial for elbow health in a program focused on improving bench-pressing strength.

SETUP: Stand normally with your arms extended toward the floor, a dumbbell in each hand, and your palms facing forward.

ACTION: Contract your biceps and curl the weights toward your shoulders. Rotate your forearms so that the palms face the floor as you lower the weights back down to the starting position. Rotate your forearms back to their original position.

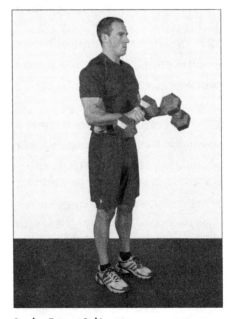

Standing Zottman Curl Lowering

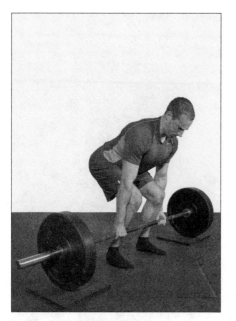

Deadlift with Bar Slightly Elevated Start

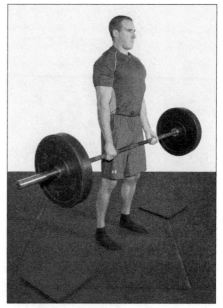

Deadlift with Bar Slightly Elevated Top

Deadlift with Bar Slightly Elevated

BENEFITS: This exercise strengthens the glutes, hamstrings, upper back, grip, and various core stabilizers. It's an excellent movement for those who aren't flexible enough to deadlift from the floor.

SETUP: The setup for this exercise is the same as the setup for the standard deadlift (see Phase 1, page 83–84), except you will elevate the plates a bit (with an aerobic step or stacked weight plates).

ACTION: This exercise is performed exactly like a standard deadlift, except the range of motion is slightly smaller.

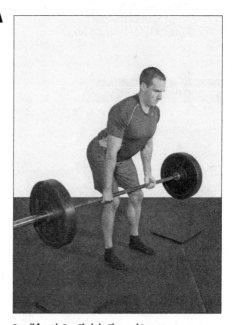

Deadlift with Bar Slightly Elevated Lowering

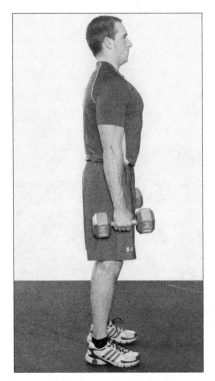

Dumbbell Reverse Lunge Start (and Finish)

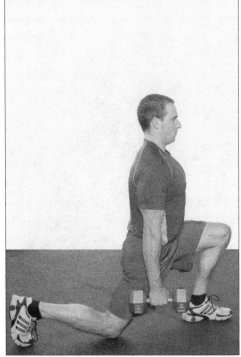

Dumbbell Reverse Lunge Middle

Dumbbell Reverse Lunge

BENEFITS: This exercise strengthens the glutes, hamstrings, quadriceps, grip, and various core stabilizers.

SETUP: Stand normally with your arms hanging at your sides and a dumbbell in each hand.

ACTION: Take a long step backward with one leg while keeping the majority of your weight on your front heel and maintaining an upright torso posture. Use the front leg to decelerate your descent and propel your body back up to the starting position. That's one rep. Complete a full set on one leg, rest, and then work the other leg (i.e., don't alternate legs from rep to rep).

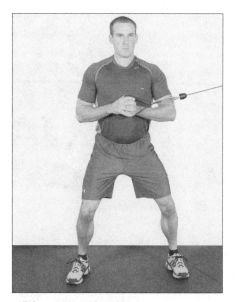

Pallof Press Start (and Finish)

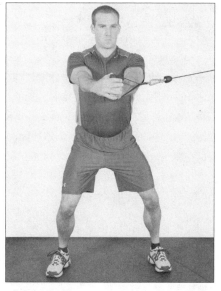

Pallof Press Middle

Pallof Press

BENEFITS: This movement, named after my friend John Pallof, a brilliant physical therapist in Massachusetts, is fantastic for training the "core" musculature's true role: resisting rotation. It is beneficial for healthy athletes and those rehabilitating injuries.

SETUP: Stand with your left side facing a cable column while holding a D-handle with both hands at chest height and your elbows flexed and hands close to your chest. Your feet should be just outside shoulder-width apart, with the knees and hips slightly bent, the chest out, and the shoulders pulled back. You'll feel the cable pulling you back toward the cable stack; your job is to resist the rotation it applies.

ACTION: Brace the core hard, and simply resist the destabilizing torque the weight stack imposes. To do a rep, extend the arms to move your hands away from your body. Hold the handle at arm's length briefly (this will be the most challenging part of the movement), and then bring the hands back in to the chest. Repeat for reps, and then switch sides. You can make this exercise more challenging by increasing the weight, keeping your feet closer together, or standing on one leg. Don't let the shoulders or hips "hike"; your upper torso should be rock solid.

Close-Grip Bench Press

BENEFITS: This exercise primarily strengthens the chest, shoulders, and triceps; the narrower grip increases the emphasis on the triceps.

SETUP: Set up the same way you do for a standard bench press (see Phase 1, page 90–91), except place your hands at shoulder width (or approximately 12 to 14 inches apart).

ACTION: Perform this exercise exactly the same way you do a standard bench press, except with a narrower grip.

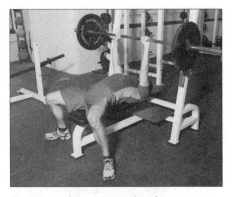

Close-Grip Bench Press Start (and Finish)

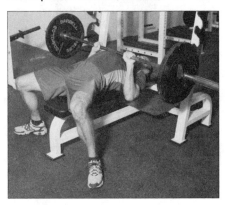

Close-Grip Bench Press Middle

Scapular Push-Up

See mobility warm-ups, page 68.

Speed Bench Press

BENEFITS: One of the best ways to get stronger is to improve the speed at which you develop force—and that's where speed exercises like this one come in. The goal here is to teach your body to be explosive with weights, not just to go through the motions.

SETUP: Set up the same way you do for a standard bench press (see Phase 1, page 90–91), but with less weight on the bar. Instead of lifting slowly against a heavier weight, you'll be focusing on lifting the weight as fast as possible with submaximal weight (you'll still want to lower the weight under control).

ACTION: Begin the same way you perform the lowering phase of a standard bench press. After the bar touches your chest, explosively push it up to the lockout position. Think "speed." Try to straighten your arms as fast as humanly possible.

Chest-Supported Row with Neutral Grip

BENEFITS: This exercise strengthens several upper-back muscles—the lats, upper/middle/lower trapezius, and rhomboids—as well as the elbow flexors (most notably, the biceps) and grip.

SETUP: Set up in a prone position on a chest-supported row apparatus and grip the handles with your palms facing each other.

ACTION: Keeping your chin tucked (avoiding neck hyperextension), pull the elbows back by retracting the shoulder blades. Don't cheat by excessively arching your back. Now extend your elbows and protract your shoulders to return to the starting position.

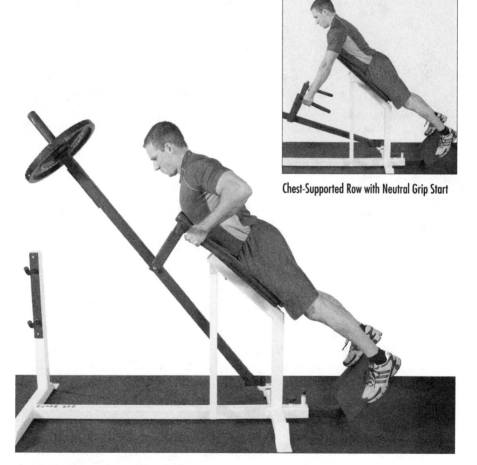

Chest-Supported Row with Neutral Grip Start

Chest-Supported Row with Neutral Grip Finish

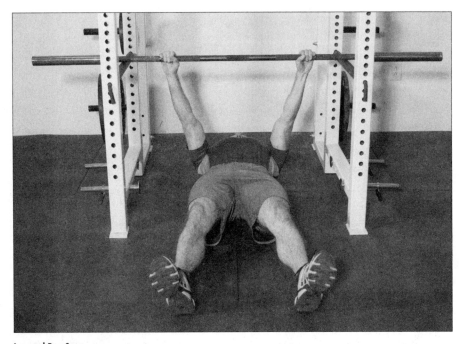

Inverted Row Start

Inverted Row

BENEFITS: This exercise strengthens several upper-back muscles—the lats, upper/middle/lower trapezius, and rhomboids—as well as the elbow flexors (most notably, the biceps) and grip.

SETUP: Set a barbell on the pins in a rack (or a Smith machine) at mid-thigh level. Lie face up on the floor under the bar with your hands positioned as if you're going to do a bench press.

ACTION: Pull yourself upward until your sternum touches the bar, and then return to the starting position. Think about pulling the shoulder blades back and down during the pulling phase. Keep your entire body in a straight line throughout this movement. Don't allow the hips to sag. There are four variations of this exercise. Here they are in order of increasing difficulty:

1. Knees bent, feet on floor
2. Knees locked, feet on floor
3. Knees locked, feet elevated on bench
4. Knees locked, feet on bench with weight plate on chest

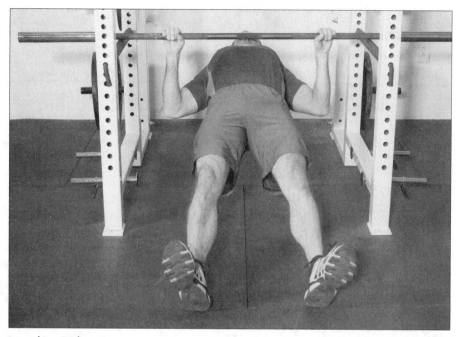

Inverted Row Finish

PHASE 2 STRENGTH-TRAINING SCHEDULE

On the next page is your four-week strength-training schedule for Phase 2. Remember to begin each session by doing one of the two warm-ups presented in Chapter 5. In each exercise involving external weight/resistance, use the highest level of weight/resistance you can lift for the designated number of repetitions with perfect form. In exercises involving no external resistance (bar rollout, etc.), simply perform the designated number of repetitions. Between sets, rest as long as necessary to perform the next set at the same level of performance, but no longer. When you see "A1" and "A2" or "B1" and "B2," etc., you should alternate between those two exercises.

PHASE 2 ENERGY WORKOUT RECOMMENDATIONS

Following are energy workout recommendations for Phase 2. Separate recommendations are provided for each of the three somatotypes discussed in Chapter 3.

PHASE 2 TRAINING SCHEDULE

	WEEK 5 HIGH	WEEK 6 MEDIUM	WEEK 7 VERY HIGH	WEEK 8 LOW
SUNDAY: REST OR ENERGY WORKOUT				
MONDAY: LOWER BODY				
Ⓐ Front Squat	(4x2)x5 10s	(5x1)x5 10s	(4x1)x6 10s	omit
Ⓑ Dumbell Step-Up	3x8 /side	3x6 /side	4x8 /side	2x6 /side (easy)
Ⓒ1 Bar Rollout	3x10	2x10	3x10	2x10
Ⓒ2 Natural Glute-Ham Raise	3x8	2x8	3x8	2x8
Ⓓ Single-Leg Squat to Box	2x10 /side	2x10 /side	2x10 /side	2x10 /side
TUESDAY: REST OR ENERGY WORKOUT				
WEDNESDAY: UPPER BODY				
Ⓐ1 Incline Barbell Press	(4x2)x5 10s	(5x1)x5 10s	(4x1)x6 10s	omit
Ⓐ2 Weighted Medium-Grip Pull-Up	(4x2)x5 10s	(5x2)x5 10s	(4x2)x6 10s	3x5 (easy)
Ⓑ1 Dumbbell Bench Press	3x8	3x6	3x8	2x6 (easy)
Ⓑ2 Head-Supported Dumbbell Row	3x8	3x6	3x8	2x6 (easy)
Ⓒ1 Cable Backhand	3x12	3x12	3x12	3x12
Ⓒ2 Standing Zottman Curl	3x10	2x10	3x10	2x10

	WEEK 5 HIGH	WEEK 6 MEDIUM	WEEK 7 VERY HIGH	WEEK 8 LOW
THURSDAY: REST OR ENERGY WORKOUT				
FRIDAY: LOWER BODY				
Ⓐ Broad Jump	5x5	5x5	6x5	omit
Ⓑ Deadlift with Bar Slightly Elevated	5x5	4x5	5x5	2x5
Ⓒ Dumbbell Reverse Lunge	3x6 /side	3x6 /side	4x6 /side	3x6 /side
Ⓓ Pallof Press	3x10 /side	3x10 /side	3x10 /side	3x10 /side
SATURDAY: UPPER BODY				
Ⓐ Speed Bench Press	10x3 @40% 1RM	8x3 @45% 1RM, then 2x3 heavy	10x3 @50% 1RM	5x3 @55% 1RM, then 1RM test
Ⓑ1 Close-Grip Bench Press	4x5	3x5	5x5	2x5
Ⓑ2 Chest-Supported Row with Neutral Grip	4x5	3x5	5x5	2x5
Ⓒ1 Inverted Row	3x10	3x10	3x10	3x10
Ⓒ2 Scapular Push-Up	3x15	3x15	3x15	3x15

Key to Notations: (4x2)x5–10s = Do five total clusters, each of which consists of four "minisets" of two reps. In this example, you'll do two reps, rest 10 seconds, do two reps, rest 10 seconds, do two reps, rest 10 seconds, and then do two reps to complete that cluster. Rest several minutes before moving to your second of five total clusters. You'll want to use approximately your five-rep max load for this particular loading scheme (others might be lighter or heavier).

5x4 = Five sets of four repetitions, and so forth.
3x30s = Three sets of 30 seconds.

Ectomorphs

TUESDAY AND THURSDAY.   Technique practice (see page 24 for a sample technique practice session) with 30 percent of one-rep max, then 20 minutes low-intensity cardio (at 60 to 70 percent of max heart rate).

Mesomorphs

IMMEDIATELY FOLLOWING EACH STRENGTH-TRAINING SESSION.   Ten minutes of low-intensity cardio (cycling, running, etc., at 60 to 70 percent of max heart rate).

TUESDAY.   Twenty minutes (excluding warm-up and cooldown) of high-intensity interval training on a 30-seconds work/60-seconds rest cycle on the elliptical trainer, bicycle, rower, or running.

THURSDAY.   Technique practice (see page 24 for a sample technique practice session) with 30 percent of one-rep max, then 20 minutes of low-intensity cardio (at 60 to 70 percent of max heart rate).

Endomorphs

IMMEDIATELY FOLLOWING EACH STRENGTH-TRAINING SESSION.   Ten minutes of low-intensity cardio (cycling, running, etc.) (at 60 to 70 percent of max heart rate).

SATURDAY.   Replace low-intensity postlifting cardio with 10 minutes of high-intensity interval training on a 30-seconds work/60-seconds rest cycle on the elliptical trainer, bicycle, rower, or running.

TUESDAY.   Twenty minutes (excluding warm-up and cooldown) of high-intensity interval training on a 45-seconds work/90-seconds rest cycle on the elliptical trainer, bicycle, rower, or running.

THURSDAY.   Technique practice (see page 24 for a sample technique practice session) with 30 percent of one-rep max, then 20 minutes of low-intensity cardio (at 60 to 70 percent of max heart rate).

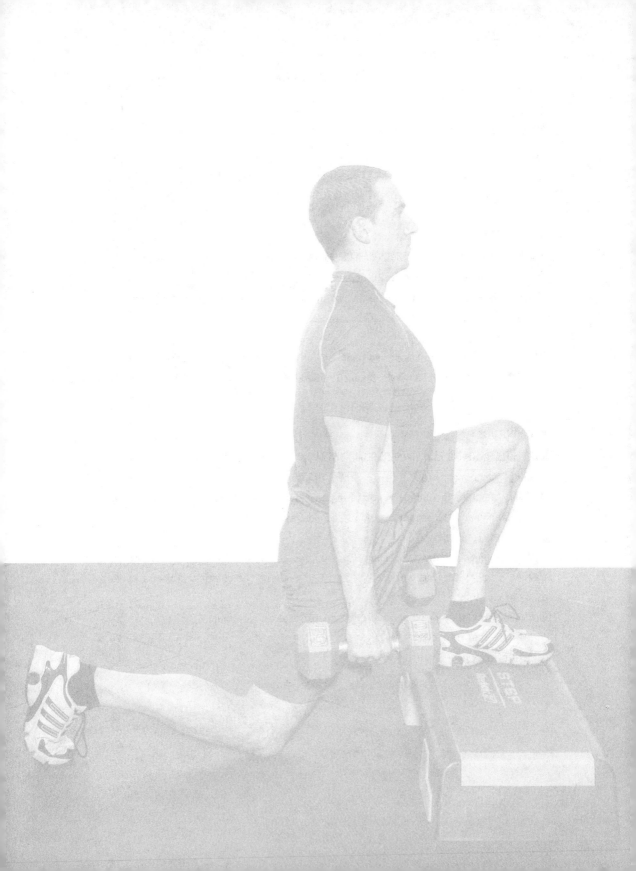

CHAPTER 8

PHASE 3: GROWTH

You've made a lot of progress in only eight weeks. But in Phase 3 you can expect your visible muscle gains and measurable strength gains to accelerate. If you've been training hard and consistently thus far, and you continue to do so in Phase 3, you will add weight to the bar throughout this next four-week period. And while most of your strength gains to this point have come from improvements in neuromuscular efficiency, in Phase 3 they will be fueled equally by gains in muscle mass. Expect to see visible growth in all of your major muscle groups.

This chapter provides all of the information you need to achieve maximum progress in Phase 3. All of the strength exercises are described and illustrated, and a detailed schedule of training sessions, which emphasize the stage system, and energy workout recommendations are given at the end of the chapter.

PHASE 3 STRENGTH EXERCISES

There are 23 strength exercises included in this phase, with almost no overlap with the preceding phases. The amount of resistance/weight you use in each exercise depends on how many repetitions per set are prescribed in a given session. As a general rule, use the highest level of resistance/weight with which you can complete the prescribed number of repetitions with perfect form. This rule does not apply to exercises that use only body weight for resistance, such as the reverse crunch. You will find specific training guidelines in the Phase 3 Strength-Training Schedule at the end of the chapter.

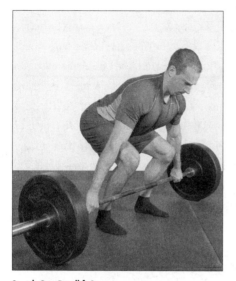

Snatch-Grip Deadlift Start

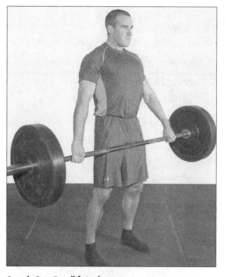

Snatch-Grip Deadlift Lockout

Snatch-Grip Deadlift

BENEFITS: This is a great movement for the glutes, hamstrings, upper back, and grip.

SETUP: The primary objective of this exercise is not using maximal weight, but making sure you perform the exercise properly. Assume a shoulder-width stance with a weighted barbell positioned on the floor just in front of your shins. Grip the bar so that your index fingers are at the rings on the barbell (well outside shoulder width). Your body weight should be on the mid foot or shifted slightly toward the heels. Lift the chest high and pull the shoulder blades back and down.

ACTION: Shift your weight to the heels and imagine pushing your heels through the floor as you explosively contract your entire posterior chain. You want the hips

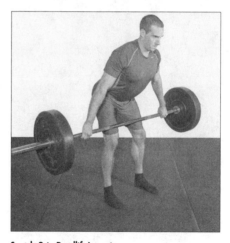

Snatch-Grip Deadlift Lowering

and shoulders to rise at the same rate. Keep your chest high and your shoulder blades tight throughout the movement; there should be little or no movement around the upper torso. Stand up fully, pause, and return to the starting position.

Front Box Squat

BENEFITS: This exercise strengthens the glutes, hamstrings, quadriceps, and various core stabilizers.

SETUP: Place a box behind you in a squat or power rack. The box height should put you at a point where the crease of your hips is just below the kneecap in the bottom position. Aside from the box element, set up the same way you set up for a standard box squat (see Phase 1, page 81).

ACTION: Brace your core, take a big gulp of air into your lungs, and sit back to the box, keeping the weight on your heels. Do not bounce off the box. Just touch it and return to the starting position with a powerful upward thrust.

Seated 90/90 Stretch

See page 65.

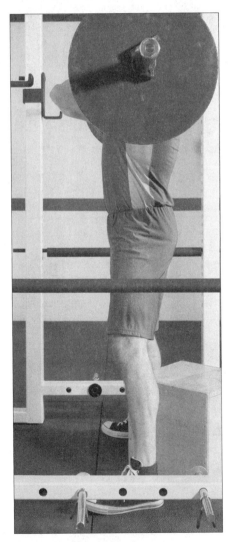

Front Box Squat Start (and Finish)

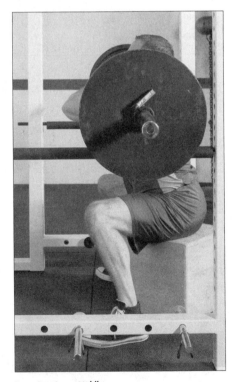

Front Box Squat Middle

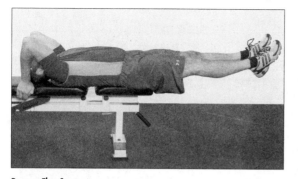

Dragon Flag Start

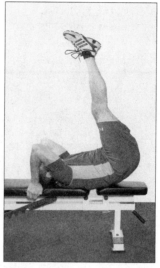

Dragon Flag Middle

Dragon Flag

BENEFITS: This movement is a progression from the reverse crunch, as it increases the challenge to the external obliques (lower abs).

SETUP: Lie face up on a bench with only the glutes and upper body supported and the legs extended straight outward in line with your torso, ankles together.

ACTION: Contract the abs to raise the legs until they form a right angle with your torso; then push the heels of your feet toward the ceiling and lift your butt off the bench slightly. Return to the starting position slowly and under control. Try to keep your hip flexors out of the movement.

Speed Deadlift

See Phase 1, pages 83–84.

Walking Dumbbell Lunge

See Phase 1, pages 86–87.

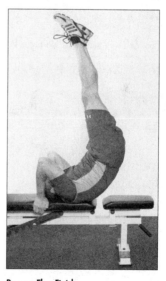

Dragon Flag Finish

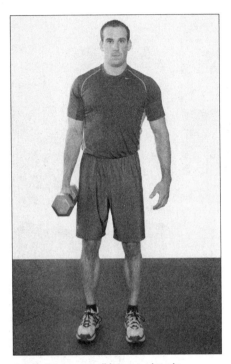

Dumbbell Suitcase Deadlift Start (and Finish)

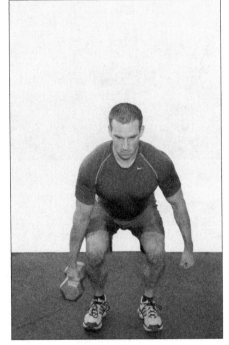

Dumbbell Suitcase Deadlift Middle

Dumbbell Suitcase Deadlift

BENEFITS: This movement is fantastic for training core stability, and specifically the ability to resist rotation. The idea is to remain "symmetrical" in spite of a significant destabilizing torque attempting to pull you out of alignment.

SETUP: Stand normally with your arms hanging at your sides and a dumbbell in one hand.

ACTION: Push your hips back and bend the knees as you do in the lowering phase of a standard deadlift. Reach the dumbbell down as close to the floor as you can get it without rounding your lower back, and then stand up again. Don't allow your torso to tilt to either side while performing this movement. You won't "feel" this movement the way you do a biceps curl or calf raise, but trust me: It's working!

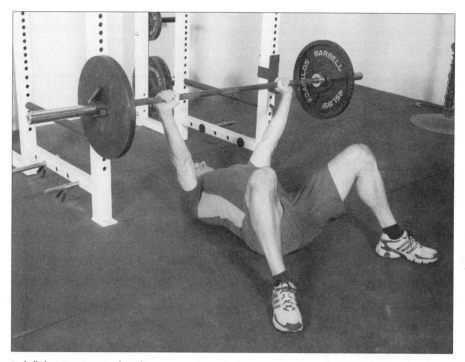

Barbell Floor Press Start (and Finish)

Barbell Floor Press

BENEFITS: This is a bench press performed on the floor. The limited range of motion will allow you to better train your lockout and reduce the load for your shoulders. You'll have less leg drive on the floor, so it becomes more upper body-focused.

SETUP: Lie face up on the floor with your arms extended toward the ceiling and a standard bench press grip on a weighted barbell.

ACTION: Lower your elbows to the floor. Don't allow the floor to absorb any of the

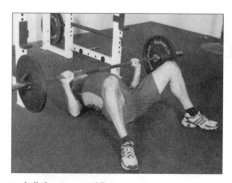

Barbell Floor Press Middle

barbell's weight through your upper arms. Allow your arms to just graze the floor, and then press the bar back toward the ceiling.

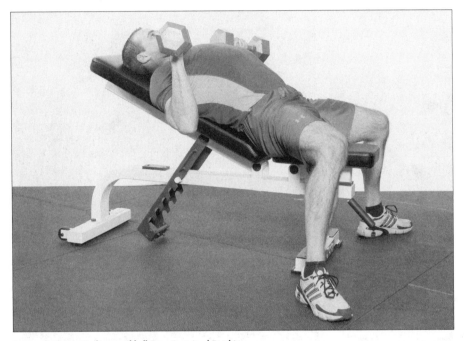

Pronated-Grip Low-Incline Dumbbell Press Start (and Finish)

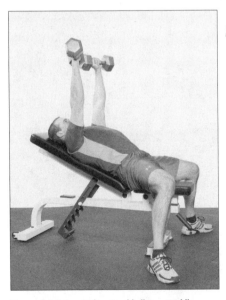

Pronated-Grip Low-Incline Dumbbell Press Middle

Pronated-Grip Low-Incline Dumbbell Press

BENEFITS: This exercise primarily strengthens the chest, shoulders, and triceps.

SETUP: Set up the same way you set up for the neutral-grip low-incline dumbbell press (see Phase 1, page 92), but use a pronated (overhand) grip instead.

ACTION: Perform this exercise the same way you do the low-incline dumbbell press with neutral grip, using a pronated grip instead.

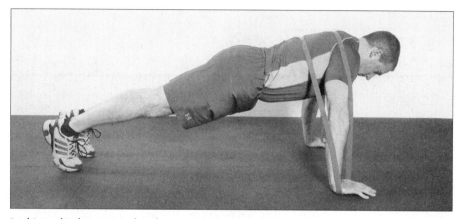

Band-Resisted Push-Up Start (and Finish)

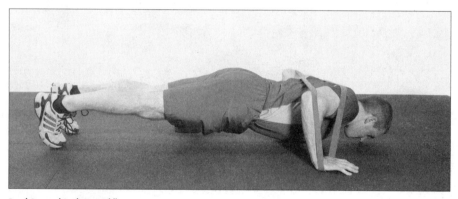

Band-Resisted Push-Up Middle

Band-Resisted Push-Up

BENEFITS: This movement provides the same benefits as the regular push-up, but there is an increased challenge to stability and lockout strength. It's an excellent progression for guys who are too strong for body weight alone on push-ups.

SETUP: Set up exactly as you would for a regular push-up (see Phase 1, page 105, but this time, you'll have a band—either a half-inch or one-inch band will do, most likely—wrapped around your upper back with the ends pressed between your palms and the floor.

ACTION: Perform this exercise the same way you do a standard push-up, but with the extra resistance provided by the band.

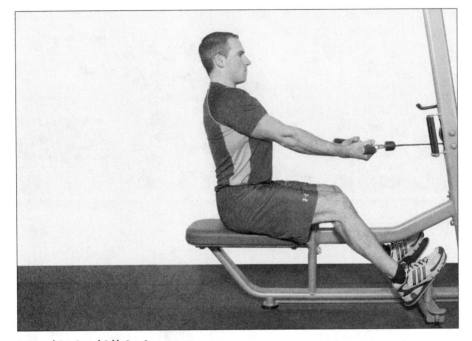

Supinated-Grip Seated Cable Row Start

Supinated-Grip Seated Cable Row

BENEFITS: This exercise strengthens several upper-back muscles—the lats, upper/middle/lower trapezius, and rhomboids—as well as the elbow flexors (most notably, the biceps) and grip.

SETUP: Sit at a cable row station with a slight bend in the knees. Grab the handle with both palms facing up and roughly shoulder-width apart. Keep the chest out, shoulders back, and eyes straight ahead so that you're sitting up tall.

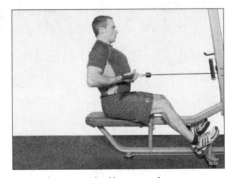

Supinated-Grip Seated Cable Row Finish

ACTION: Pull your shoulder blades back and down, bend your elbows, and draw the handle to your stomach. Think "shoulder blades back and down" as you lift the weight. Return to the starting position.

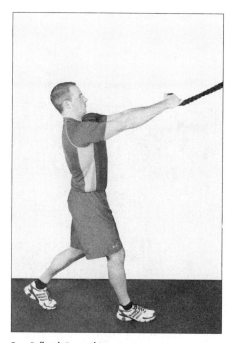

Face Pull with External Rotation Start

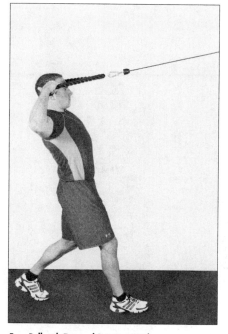

Face Pull with External Rotation Finish

Face Pull with External Rotation

BENEFITS: This exercise strengthens several upper-back muscles—the lats, upper/middle/lower trapezius, and rhomboids—as well as the elbow flexors (most notably, the biceps) and grip. The inclusion of extra external rotation in the movement makes it an even better exercise for preventing shoulder problems.

SETUP: Set up a pulley with the rope attachment just above forehead level. Stand facing the pulley in a split stance and hold the rope with a neutral grip (palms and face in). Your arms are extended straight out in front of you with the hands slightly above shoulder height.

ACTION: Pull the center of the rope attachment toward your forehead by retracting the shoulder blades and forcing the elbows out (not down). As the rope approaches your face, your shoulder blades should be pulled back and down, with the chest high and your hands coming even with your ears. You should feel the resistance in your mid back and in the back of your shoulders.

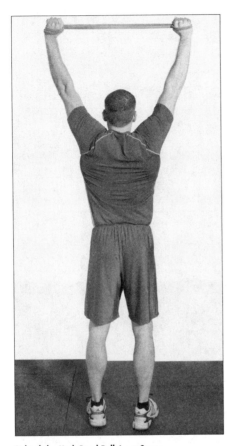

Behind-the-Neck Band Pull-Apart Start

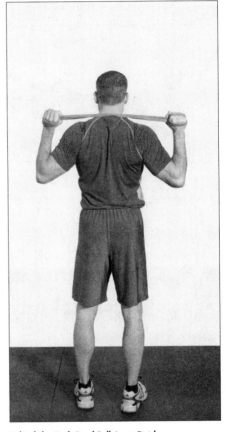

Behind-the-Neck Band Pull-Apart Finish

Behind-the-Neck Band Pull-Apart

BENEFITS: This exercise strengthens the lower trapezius muscles, which are very important for adequate scapular upward rotation and overall shoulder health.

SETUP: Stand with your arms extended straight overhead and grasp a short resistance band with your hands at shoulder width and palms facing forward.

ACTION: By pulling the shoulder blades back and down and flexing the elbows, lower the band to a position behind your neck. The band will stretch several inches as this action is performed. You'll feel the effort in the muscles at the base of your shoulder blades. Be careful not to let your chin protrude forward; keep it tucked. Return to the starting position.

Speed Free Squat: Medium Stance

BENEFITS: This exercise strengthens the glutes, hamstrings, quadriceps, and several core stabilizers. It's always a good idea to incorporate some free squatting in a program that includes a lot of box squatting so that you don't become overly dependent on the box.

SETUP: Stand with a weighted barbell resting on your upper back, your hands holding it in place, and your feet positioned just slightly farther apart than shoulder-width.

ACTION: Take a big gulp of air into your belly, brace your core, and squat back slowly and under control until your thighs are parallel to the floor. Thrust powerfully upward to a standing position. Think "speed" and "explosion," as though you're trying not just to stand but to jump.

Rack Pull from Kneecaps
See Phase 1, Page 100.

Wall Ankle Mobilization
See page 57.

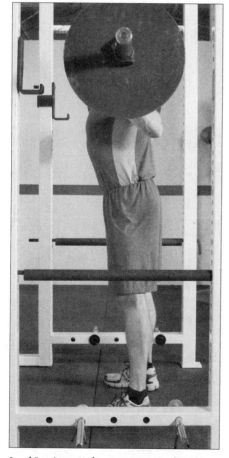

Speed Free Squat: Medium Stance Start (and Finish)

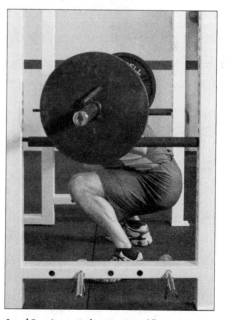

Speed Free Squat: Medium Stance Middle

Dumbbell Reverse Lunge: Front Foot Elevated

BENEFITS: This exercise utilizes an increased range of motion to further strengthen the glutes, hamstrings, quadriceps, grip, and various core stabilizers.

SETUP: Stand on a four- to six-inch step with your arms resting at your sides and a dumbbell in each hand.

ACTION: Take a big step backward with one leg and bend both knees until the knee of the back leg grazes the floor; then thrust powerfully upward and forward off the rear foot and return to the starting position. Be sure to maintain an upright torso posture throughout the movement. Complete the designated number of reps with one leg, rest, and then work the opposite leg.

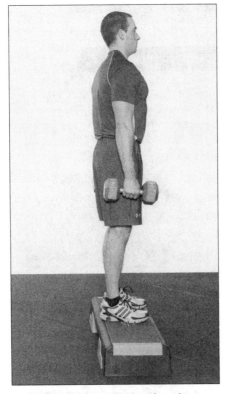

Dumbbell Reverse Lunge: Front Foot Elevated Start (and Finish)

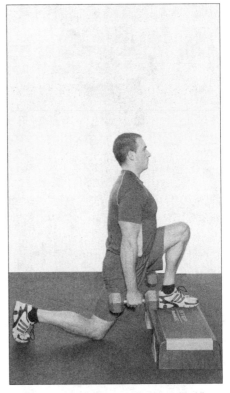

Dumbbell Reverse Lunge: Front Foot Elevated Middle

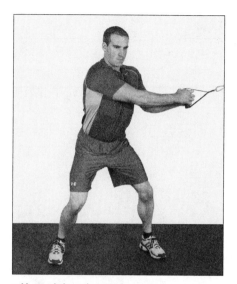

Cable Wood Chop: Chest Height Start

Cable Wood Chop: Chest Height Finish

Cable Wood Chop: Chest Height

BENEFITS: This exercise is fantastic for training rotation, which is an important movement pattern in our daily lives. We want to condition ourselves to rotate in only certain places (not the lumbar spine), and the first two phases of this program have prepared you to do this movement, which trains proper rotation, in the third phase. The cable wood chop also strengthens dozens of core stabilizers.

SETUP: Stand with your left side facing a cable column while holding a D-handle with both hands, your arms fully extended at chest level, and your torso rotated to the left so that your arms are pointing toward the cable column. Your feet should be just outside shoulder-width apart, with the knees and hips slightly bent, the chest out, and shoulders pulled back.

ACTION: Brace your abs hard and pivot at your hips and thoracic spine/shoulders in order to rotate as if you were swinging a baseball bat at chest height. You don't want any of the rotation to occur at your lumbar (lower) spine, so if you're feeling this in your lower back, you're doing it incorrectly. In this case, take the weight down and practice the technique. Return under control to the starting position. The arms should be just short of lockout for the duration of each rep. After completing a full set, turn around and chop in the opposite direction.

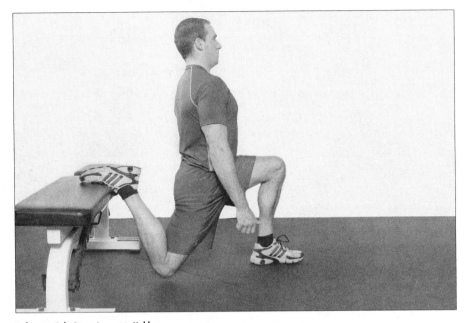

Bulgarian Split-Squat Isometric Hold

Bulgarian Split-Squat Isometric Hold

BENEFITS: Like all single-leg movements, this one strengthens the glutes, hamstrings, quadriceps, and hip adductors. But with its isometric hold (i.e., a muscle contraction in a fixed position), this one also provides a great stretch for the hip flexors. Effectively, it's an active flexibility exercise.

SETUP: Position a bench roughly three feet behind you. Stand normally with your arms hanging at your sides.

ACTION: Step backward onto the bench with one foot. Break at the knee of the forward leg and lower yourself down into a split-squat position. In the bottom position, the knee of your trailing leg should be just short of touching the floor, with the torso upright and shoulders pulled back. You'll feel a great stretch on the front of the hip and thigh of the trailing leg. Your weight should be almost completely on the mid-foot of the forward leg with the toe of the back foot just helping you to maintain balance.

Hold this position for the prescribed amount of time. Actively contract all of the involved muscles for the entire duration for the hold. Think "glutes and hamstrings active, hip flexors relaxed." Many people literally fall over toward the end of a set. Others tap out quickly because the fantastic stretch on the back leg takes them out of their comfort zone.

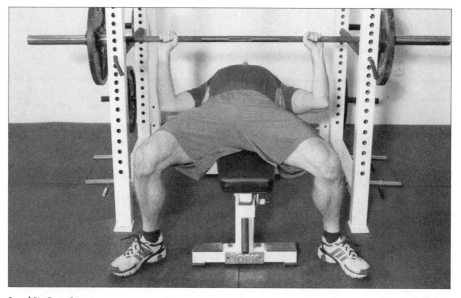

Speed Pin Press Start

Speed Pin Press

BENEFITS: This exercise teaches your body to be explosive with weights, rather than just going through the motions. It is an excellent movement to develop bottom-end strength on the bench press.

SETUP: Set up a bench inside a power rack so that the safety pins are about two inches above your chest when you're lying on the bench in your normal bench-press starting position.

ACTION: This movement is similar to a two-board press (see Phase 4, page 163), but you will perform the lifting segment explosively, and instead of using boards, you'll rest the bar briefly on the pins in the power rack. Weight the bar so that you can push it away from

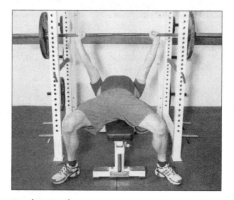

Speed Pin Finish

your chest at twice your normal bench-press tempo. Lower the bar slowly and under control. Otherwise, follow all of the same cues that apply to the standard bench press, including concentrating on keeping your upper back tight in the bottom position.

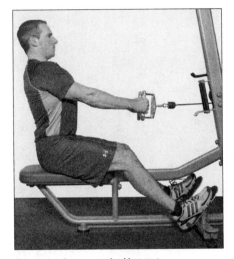

Close, Neutral-Grip Seated Cable Row Start

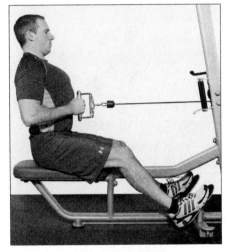

Close, Neutral-Grip Seated Cable Row Finish

Close, Neutral-Grip Seated Cable Row

BENEFITS: This exercise strengthens several upper-back muscles—the lats, upper/middle/lower trapezius, and rhomboids—as well as the elbow flexors (most notably, the biceps) and grip.

SETUP: Sit at a cable row station with a slight bend in the knees. Grab the handle with both hands facing each other and less than shoulder-width apart. Keep the chest out, shoulders back, and eyes straight ahead so that you're sitting up tall.

ACTION: Pull your shoulder blades back and down, bend your elbows, and draw the handle to your stomach. Think "shoulder blades back and down" as you lift the weight. Return to the starting position.

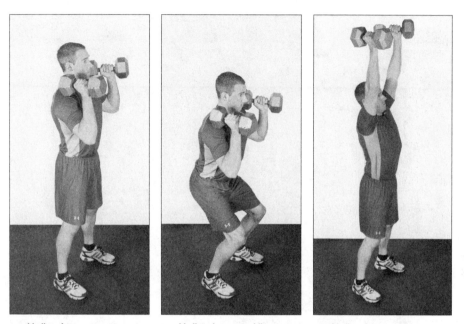

Dumbbell Push Press Start   Dumbbell Push Press Middle   Dumbbell Push Press Finish

Dumbbell Push Press

BENEFITS: This exercise strengthens the shoulders, triceps, and several core stabilizers.

SETUP: Stand with a dumbbell in each hand and your elbows fully flexed so the weights are at your shoulders. Your palms are facing each other and your feet are shoulder-width apart. Before you begin, draw a deep breath and hold it, and at the same time draw your belly button toward your spine. This position will tighten the muscles around your spine and aid the transfer of force from your legs to your arms in the explosive movement that follows.

ACTION: Bend your knees and lower yourself into a quarter squat. Immediately reverse this movement, powerfully straightening your legs and hips. As soon as you're once again fully upright, press the dumbbells straight overhead. The idea is to use the upward momentum created by straightening your legs to assist your shoulders and arms in pushing the dumbbells toward the ceiling. This momentum allows you to lift more weight than you could with a standard shoulder press. To complete the movement, lower the dumbbells back down to your shoulders.

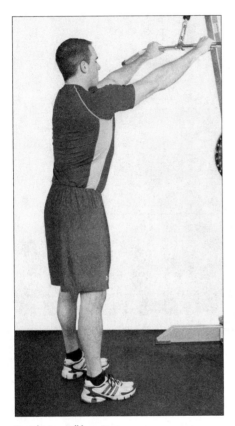

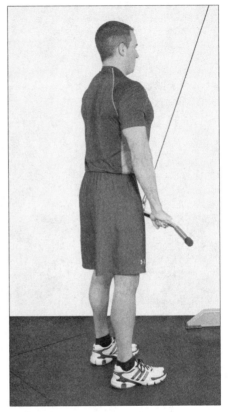

Straight-Arm Pulldown Start   **Straight-Arm Pulldown Finish**

Straight-Arm Pulldown

BENEFITS: This is another movement to strengthen the lower trapezius and keep the shoulders healthy.

SETUP: Stand facing a cable column or pulldown machine with a straight-bar attachment. Grasp the bar with a pronated (palms-down) grip and your arms extended straight in front of you with the bar at shoulder height.

ACTION: Keeping your torso upright and initiating the movement with your shoulder blades and upper arms, pull the bar down until it touches your upper thighs while keeping the wrists and elbows straight. When this exercise is performed correctly, you'll feel it in your mid back, right at the base of your shoulder blades.

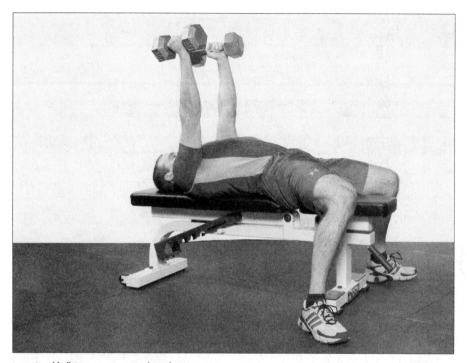

Lying Dumbbell Extension Start (and Finish)

Lying Dumbbell Extension

BENEFITS: This movement provides some extra volume to strengthen the triceps, which are heavily recruited with power-lifting-style bench pressing.

SETUP: Lie face up on the floor or a bench with your arms extended straight overhead and a dumbbell in each hand, palms facing each other.

ACTION: Bend the elbows and lower the dumbbells back toward your ears while keeping the elbows pointed toward the ceiling. When you get to the end of

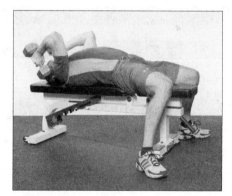

Lying Dumbbell Extension Middle

the range of motion, press the dumbbells back to the starting position with the strength of your triceps.

PHASE 3 TRAINING SCHEDULE

		WEEK 9 HIGH	WEEK 10 MEDIUM	WEEK 11 VERY HIGH	WEEK 12 LOW
SUNDAY: REST OR ENERGY WORKOUT					
MONDAY: LOWER BODY					
A1	Snatch-Grip Deadlift (Weeks 9, 10); Front Box Squat (Weeks 11, 12)	3x3, 2x5	4x2, 2x4	4x3, 2x5	2x2, 1x4
A2	Seated 90/90 Stretch	15s /side	15s /side	15s /side	15s /side
B	Speed Deadlift	8x1 @60% 1RM	8x1 @65% 1RM	10x1 @70% 1RM	omit
C	Walking Dumbbell Lunge	3x7, 1x10 /side	3x7, 1x10 /side	3x7, 1x10 /side	2x7, 1x10 /side
D1	Dragon Flag	3x12	3x12	3x12	3x12
D2	Dumbbell Suitcase Deadlift	3x10	3x10	3x10	3x10
TUESDAY: REST OR ENERGY WORKOUT					
WEDNESDAY: UPPER BODY					
A	Barbell Floor Press (Weeks 9, 10); Pronated-Grip Low-Incline Dumbbell Press (Weeks 11, 12)	3x3 2x5	4x2 2x4	4x3 2x5	2x2 1x4
B1	Band-Resisted Push-Up	3x7, 1x10	3x7, 1x10	3x7, 1x10	2x7, 1x10
B2	Supinated-Grip Seated Cable Row	3x7, 1x10	3x7, 1x10	3x7, 1x10	2x7, 1x10
C1	Face Pull w/External Rotation	3x10	3x10	3x10	3x10
C2	Behind-the-Neck Band Pull-Apart	3x12 /side	3x12 /side	3x12 /side	3x12 /side

		WEEK 9 HIGH	WEEK 10 MEDIUM	WEEK 11 VERY HIGH	WEEK 12 LOW
THURSDAY: REST OR ENERGY WORKOUT					
FRIDAY: LOWER BODY					
A	Speed Free Squat: Medium Stance	10x2 @50% 1RM	8x2 @55% 1RM, Then 2x2 heavy	10x2 @60% 1RM	5x2 @55% 1RM, Then 2x2 heavy
B1	Rack Pull from Kneecaps	3x5, 2x7	2x5, 1x7	3x5, 2x7	2x5, 1x7
B2	Wall Ankle Mobilization	4x8 /side	3x8 /side	4x8 /side	3x8 /side
C	Dumbbell Reverse Lunge: Front Foot Elevated	3x5, 1x7	2x5, 1x7	3x5, 1x7	2x5, 1x7
D1	Cable Wood Chop: Chest Height	3x10 /side	2x10 /side	3x10 /side	omit
D2	Bulgarian Split-Squat Isometric Hold	2x30s /side	2x30s /side	3x30s /side	1x30s /side
SATURDAY: UPPER BODY					
A	Speed Pin Press	10x3 @50% 1RM	8x3 @55% 1RM, Then 2x2 heavy	10x3 @60% 1RM	5x3 @55% 1RM, Then 2x2 heavy
B1	Close, Neutral-Grip Seated Cable Row	3x5, 2x7	3x5, 1x7	3x5, 2x7	2x5, 1x7
B2	Dumbbell Push Press	3x5, 1x7	3x5, 1x7	3x5, 2x7	2x5, 1x7
C1	Straight-Arm Pulldown	3x12	3x12	3x12	3x12
C2	Lying Dumbbell Extension	2x10	2x10	3x10	omit

Key to Notations: 3x3, 2x5 = Three sets of three repetitions, then two sets of five repetitions (with slightly less weight).   3x12= Three sets of 12 repetitions. 2x30s = Two sets of 30 seconds.

PHASE 3 STRENGTH-TRAINING SCHEDULE

Here is your four-week strength-session schedule for Phase 3. Remember to begin each session by doing one of the two warm-ups presented in Chapter 5. In each exercise involving external weight/resistance, use the highest level of weight/resistance you can lift for the designated number of repetitions with perfect form. In exercises involving no external resistance (dragon flag, etc.), simply perform the designated number of repetitions. Between sets, rest as long as necessary to perform the next set at the same level of performance, but no longer. When you see "A1" and "A2" or "B1" and "B2," etc., you should alternate between those two exercises.

PHASE 3 ENERGY WORKOUT RECOMMENDATIONS

Following are energy workout recommendations for Phase 3. Separate recommendations are provided for each of the three somatotypes discussed in Chapter 3.

Ectomorphs

TUESDAY AND THURSDAY. Technique practice (see page 24 for a sample technique practice session) with 30 percent of one-rep max, then 20 minutes of low-intensity cardio (at 60 to 70 percent of max heart rate).

Mesomorphs

IMMEDIATELY FOLLOWING EACH STRENGTH-TRAINING SESSION. Ten minutes of low-intensity cardio (cycling, running, etc., at 60 to 70 percent of max heart rate).

TUESDAY. Twenty minutes (excluding warm-up and cooldown) of high-intensity interval training on a 20-seconds work/40-seconds rest cycle on the elliptical trainer, bicycle, rower, or running.

THURSDAY. Technique practice (see page 24 for a sample technique practice session) with 30 percent of one-rep max, then 20 minutes of low-intensity cardio (at 60 to 70 percent of max heart rate).

Endomorphs

IMMEDIATELY FOLLOWING EACH STRENGTH-TRAINING SESSION. Ten minutes of low-intensity cardio (cycling, running, etc., at 60 to 70 percent of max heart rate).

SATURDAY.   Replace low-intensity postlifting cardio with 10 minutes of high-intensity interval training on a 30-seconds work/60-seconds rest cycle on the elliptical trainer, bicycle, rower, or running.

TUESDAY.   Twenty minutes (excluding warm-up and cooldown) of high-intensity interval training on a 45-seconds work/90-seconds rest cycle on the elliptical trainer, bicycle, rower, or running.

THURSDAY.   Technique practice (see page 24 for a sample technique practice session) with 30 percent of one-rep max, then 20 minutes of low-intensity cardio (at 60 to 70 percent of max heart rate).

CHAPTER 9

PHASE 4: PEAK

Phase 4 is my favorite phase of the Maximum Strength Program, not only because it culminates in Moving Day—your chance to prove just how far you've come in only 16 weeks—but also because it emphasizes single-repetition sets using loads in excess of 90 percent of one-repetition maximum (1RM), the Holy Grail of maximum strength development. This chapter provides all of the information you need to achieve the best possible results on Moving Day. All of the strength exercises are described and illustrated, and a detailed schedule of strength-training sessions and energy workout recommendations are also provided. In the final section of the chapter I will present brief instructions for Moving Day and provide space to record your results.

PHASE 4 STRENGTH EXERCISES

There is somewhat more overlap in strength exercise selection between this phase and the preceding phases, but there is still plenty of new stuff. Phase 4 features 21 strength exercises in total. The amount of resistance/weight you use in each exercise depends on how many repetitions per set are prescribed in a given session. As a general rule, use the highest level of resistance/weight with which you can complete the prescribed number of repetitions with perfect form. This rule does not apply to exercises that use only body weight for resistance, such as the reverse crunch. You will find specific training guidelines in the Phase 4 Strength-Training Schedule at the end of the chapter.

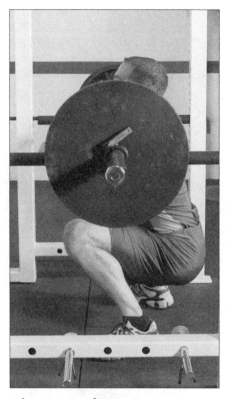

Anderson Front Squat from Pins Start

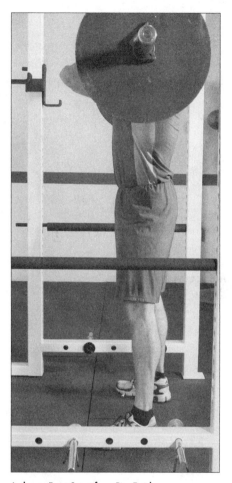

Anderson Front Squat from Pins Finish

Anderson Front Squat from Pins

BENEFITS: This movement is great for developing explosive strength—otherwise known as rate of force development. It strengthens the quadriceps, glutes, hamstrings, and several core stabilizers.

SETUP: Set up the same way you set up for a standard front squat (see Phase 1, page 98), but insert pins at the bottom position in a power rack.

ACTION: Perform this exercise the same way you do a standard front squat, but when you reach the bottom of a rep, rest the barbell on the pins for one second, and then explode back to the starting position.

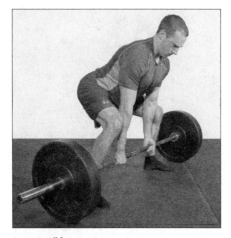

Sumo Deadlift Start

Sumo Deadlift

BENEFITS: This exercise strengthens the glutes, hamstrings, adductors (inner thighs), quadriceps, upper back, grip, and various core stabilizers.

SETUP: Position a weighted barbell on the floor. Stand in a very wide stance with your shins almost touching the bar; lower your butt toward the floor, and grab onto the bar with both hands, positioned at shoulder width or slightly closer, using an overhand or split grip. Your arms are fully extended and your chest is as high as you can get it from this position.

ACTION: Contract your entire posterior chain and stand upright. Lock out by re-tracting your shoulder blades. Note that you'll need to experiment with your stance width in this exercise to find the position that's most comfortable; some people like to go considerably wider than others.

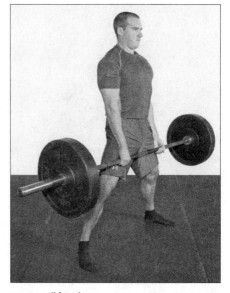

Sumo Deadlift Lockout

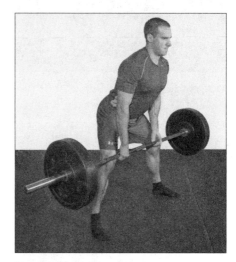

Sumo Deadlift Lowering

Speed Deadlift

See Phase 1, pages 83–84.

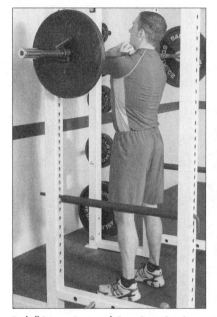 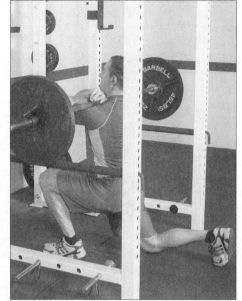

Barbell Reverse Lunge with Front-Squat Grip Start (and Finish)

Barbell Reverse Lunge with Front-Squat Grip Middle

Barbell Reverse Lunge with Front-Squat Grip

BENEFITS: This movement combines the front squat with the dumbbell reverse lunge, but it's harder than the latter because the resistance is a barbell in the front-squat position. Because you are moving your center of gravity upward, farther away from your base of support, the balance challenge becomes more significant.

SETUP: Set up the same way you set up for a front squat (see Phase 1, page 98).

ACTION: Take a backward step with one leg and bend both knees until the knee of the back leg grazes the floor. The majority of your weight should be kept on the heel of the front leg. Push through that heel to use your hamstrings and glutes to return to the starting position. Try to minimize pushing from the back leg. Complete the designated number of repetitions with the same leg, rest, and then work the other leg.

Pallof Press

See Phase 2, page 125.

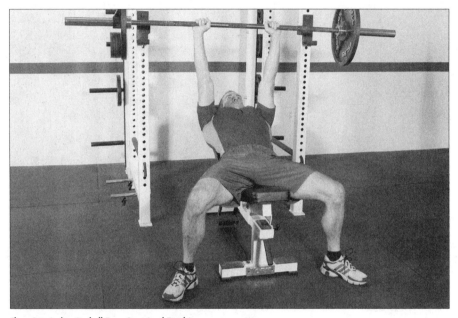

Close-Grip Incline Barbell Press Start (and Finish)

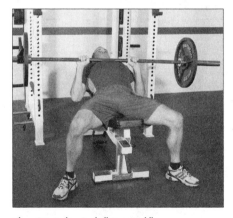

Close-Grip Incline Barbell Press Middle

Close-Grip Incline Barbell Press

BENEFITS: This exercise primarily strengthens the chest, shoulders, and triceps, although the narrower grip increases the emphasis on the triceps relative to the standard incline dumbbell press.

SETUP: Set up the same way you set up for a standard incline barbell press (see Phase 2, page 118), but position your hands only 12 to 14 inches apart.

ACTION: Perform this exercise the same way you do the standard incline barbell press.

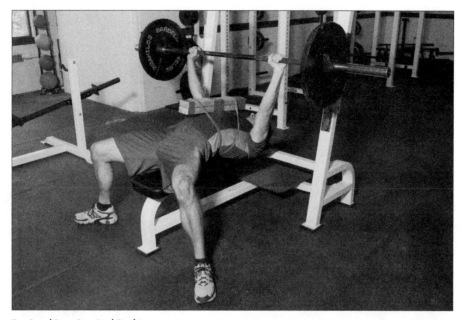

Two-Board Press Start (and Finish)

Two-Board Press

BENEFITS: This is a partial range-of-motion bench press that helps you lock out harder and get accustomed to using heavier weights. It's also good for deloading the shoulders a bit.

SETUP: This exercise requires two two-inch by four-inch slabs of wood taped together or a thick phone book. Place the boards on your chest during the exercise to limit your range of motion. It's generally best to have a partner hold the boards, but you can also get away with wrapping a miniband around your torso to hold the boards in place, or with simply sliding them under your shirt.

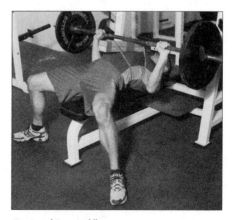

Two-Board Press Middle

ACTION: Perform this exercise the same way you do the regular bench press (see Phase 1, page 90), but with less range of motion, thanks to the boards.

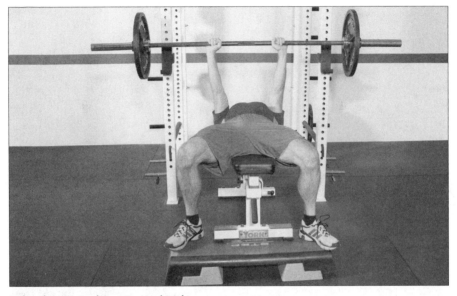

Decline Close-Grip Bench Press Start (and Finish)

Decline Close-Grip Bench Press

BENEFITS: Generally speaking, decline pressing is easier on the shoulders than flat and incline pressing, so it's a great inclusion when you want to move some big weights while giving the shoulders a break.

SETUP: Set up the same way you set up for a standard bench press (see Phase 1, page 90), but use a decline bench. If you don't have a dedicated decline bench, you can simply elevate the front end of a bench and perform the exercise in a power rack (as pictured).

ACTION: Perform this exercise the same way you perform a standard bench press.

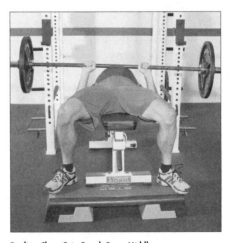

Decline Close-Grip Bench Press Middle

The only difference is that you will not be able to involve your legs from the decline position.

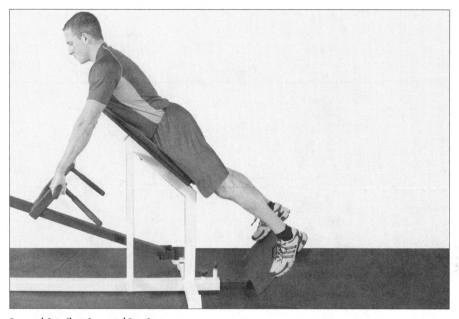

Pronated-Grip Chest-Supported Row Start

Pronated-Grip Chest-Supported Row

BENEFITS: This exercise strengthens several upper-back muscles—the lats, upper/middle/lower trapezius, and rhomboids—as well as the elbow flexors (most notably, the biceps) and grip.

SETUP: Set up on a T-bar row station and grasp the handles with your palms facing the floor.

ACTION: Retract your shoulder blades, bend your elbows, and pull the handles toward your body. Keep your body as straight as possible, with the chest pressed tight against the pad and the upper back doing the brunt of the work. Keep the chin tucked, and hold the shoulder blades back for a count of one at the top of each rep.

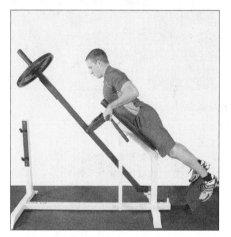

Pronated-Grip Chest-Supported Row Finish

Scapular Wall Slide

See page 69.

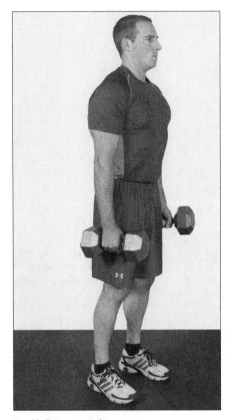

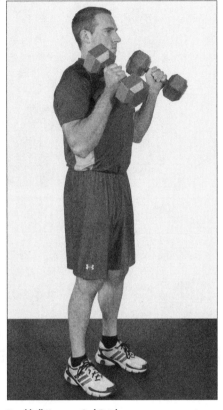

Dumbbell Hammer Curl Start   Dumbbell Hammer Curl Finish

Dumbbell Hammer Curl

BENEFITS: This exercise strengthens the biceps, and two biceps muscles in particular: the brachioradialis and brachialis.

SETUP: Stand normally with your arms relaxed at your sides, a dumbbell in each hand, and your palms facing each other.

ACTION: Contract your biceps and curl the weights toward your shoulders. Return to the starting position.

Box Squat

See Phase 1, pages 81–82.

Natural Glute-Ham Raise

See Phase 2, page 115.

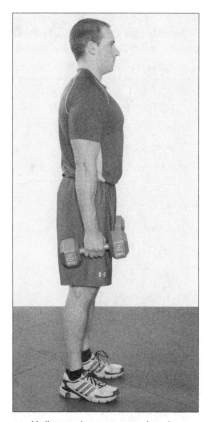

Dumbbell Forward Lunge Start (and Finish)

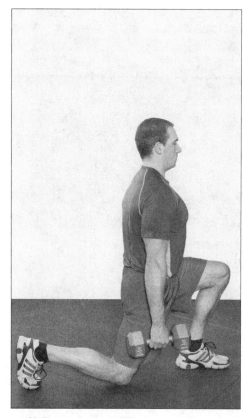

Dumbbell Forward Lunge Middle

Single-Leg Squat (Pistol) to Box

See Phase 2, page 116 (but do your best to get deeper this month!).

Dumbbell Forward Lunge

BENEFITS: This exercise strengthens the glutes, hamstrings, quadriceps, grip, and various core stabilizers.

SETUP: Stand normally with your arms re-laxed at your sides and a dumbbell in each hand.

ACTION: Take a long step forward with one leg while maintaining an upright torso posture. Use the heel of the front leg to decelerate your descent. Bend both knees until the knee of your trailing leg grazes the floor, and then thrust backward off the heel of your forward foot to return to the starting position. Continue lunging with the same leg until you've completed the designated number of repetitions; then rest and work the other leg.

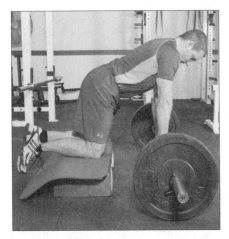

Bar Rollout: Knees on Four-Inch Box Start (and Finish)

Bar Rollout: Knees on Four-Inch Box

BENEFITS: This exercise strengthens several key core stabilizers, most notably the rectus abdominus and lats.

SETUP: Set up the same way you set up for the standard bar rollout (see Phase 2, page 114), but position a four-inch box under your knees to increase the range of motion.

ACTION: Perform this exercise the same way you do the standard bar rollout, but with your knees elevated.

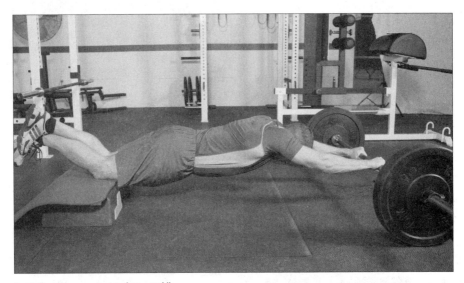

Bar Rollout: Knees on Four-Inch Box Middle

Speed Bench Press

See Phase 2, page 126.

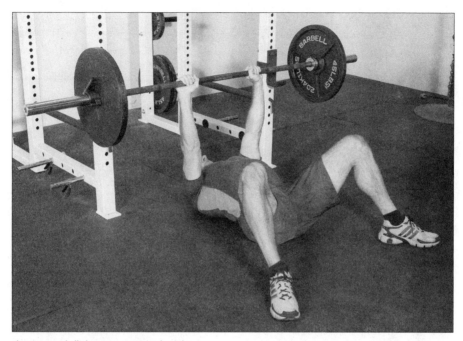

Close-Grip Barbell Floor Press Start (and Finish)

Close-Grip Barbell Floor Press

BENEFITS: This exercise strengthens the chest, shoulders, and triceps, with particular emphasis on the triceps, thanks to the limited range of motion and close grip.

SETUP: Set up the same way you set up for the standard barbell floor press (see Phase 3, page 139), but position your hands only 12 to 14 inches apart.

ACTION: Perform this exercise the same way you do the standard floor press, but with a narrow grip.

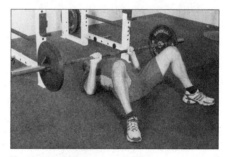

Close-Grip Barbell Floor Press Middle

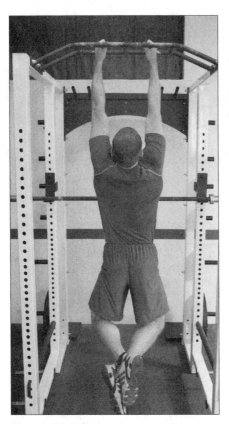

Neutral-Grip Pull-Up Start

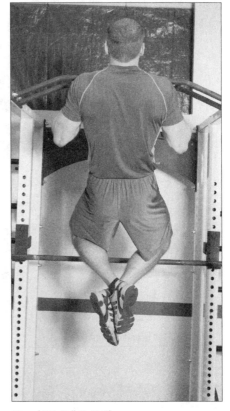

Neutral-Grip Pull-Up Finish

Neutral-Grip Pull-Up

BENEFIT: This exercise strengthens the lats, elbow flexors (including the biceps), and grip, plus several core stabilizers.

SETUP: Set up the same way you set up for the medium-grip pull-up (see Phase 2, page 117), but with your palms facing each other.

ACTION: Perform this exercise the same you do you the medium-grip pull-up, but with a neutral grip.

One-Arm Dumbbell Row

See Phase 1, page 106.

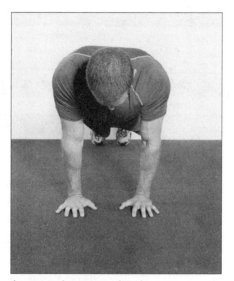

Close-Grip Push-Up Start (and Finish)

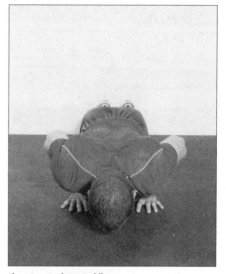

Close-Grip Push-Up Middle

Close-Grip Push-Up

BENEFIT: This variation of the push-up is another means of challenging the triceps' ability to support the working pecs, and strong triceps make for a big bench press! If the standard version of this exercise is too easy, you can always wrap a band around your back (as you did in Phase 2) to increase the difficulty.

SETUP: The setup is identical to that of the standard push-up (see Phase 1, page 105), but your hands will only be four to five inches apart.

ACTION: Perform this exercise the same way you do a standard push-up, but with the elbows staying closer to your sides during the movement.

PHASE 4 TRAINING SCHEDULE

	WEEK 13 HIGH	WEEK 14 MEDIUM	WEEK 15 VERY HIGH	WEEK 16 LOW
SUNDAY: REST OR ENERGY WORKOUT				
MONDAY: LOWER BODY				
A Anderson Front Squat from Pins (Weeks 1, 2); Sumo Deadlift (Week 3)	7 singles > 90%	5 singles > 90%	9 singles > 90%	omit
B Speed Deadlift	8x1 @60% 1RM	8x1 @65% 1RM	8x1 @70% 1RM	omit
C Barbell Reverse Lunge with Front-Squat Grip	4x8 /side	3x8 /side	4x8 /side	2x8 /side (easy)
D Pallof Press	3x8 /side	3x8 /side	3x8 /side	3x8 /side
TUESDAY: REST OR ENERGY WORKOUT				
WEDNESDAY: UPPER BODY				
A Close-Grip Incline Press (Weeks 13, 14); Two-Board Press (Weeks 15, 16)	7 singles > 90%	5 singles > 90%	9 singles > 90%	omit *
B1 Decline Close-Grip Bench Press	4x8	3x8	4x8	2x8
B2 Chest-Supported Row with Pronated Grip	4x8	3x8	4x8	2x8
C1 Scapular Wall Slide	3x12	3x12	3x12	3x12
C2 Dumbbell Hammer Curl	3x12	3x12	3x12	3x12

* During Week 16, perform this session on Tuesday.

Key to Notations: 7 singles > 90 percent = Seven sets of one rep. You shouldn't "count" a set until it feels as if it is heavier than 90 percent of the weight you can barely get for one rep.

4x8 = Four sets of eight repetitions.

	WEEK 13 HIGH	WEEK 14 MEDIUM	WEEK 15 VERY HIGH	WEEK 16 LOW
THURSDAY: REST OR ENERGY WORKOUT				
FRIDAY: LOWER BODY				
A Box Squat	10x2 @50% 1RM	8x2 @55% 1RM, Then 2x2 heavy	12x2 @60% 1RM	omit session during week 16
B Natural Glute-Ham Raise	4x5	3x5	4x5	
C Dumbbell Forward Lunge	3x6 /side	3x5 /side	4x6 /side	
D1 Single-Leg Squat (Pistols) to Box (lower this month)	3x10	3x10	3x10	
D2 Bar Rollout: Knees on Four-Inch Box	3x12	3x12	3x12	
SATURDAY: UPPER BODY				
A Speed Bench Press	10x3 @50% 1RM	8x3 @55% 1RM, Then 2x2 heavy	10x3 @60% 1RM	** Broad Jump Test
B1 Close-Grip Barbell Floor Press	4x5 2x7	3x5 1x7	4x5 2x7	1RM Squat Test
B2 Neutral-Grip Pull-Up	4x5	3x5	4x5	1RM Bench Test
C1 One-Arm Dumbbell Row	3x10	2x10	3x10	1RM Deadlift Test
C2 Close-Grip Push-Up	3x10	2x10	3x10	3RM Chin-Up Test

** MOVING DAY! Perform this session on the Final Saturday of Week 16.

PHASE 4 STRENGTH-TRAINING SCHEDULE

On the previous page is your four-week strength-training schedule for Phase 4. Remember to begin each session by doing one of the two warm-ups presented in Chapter 5. In each exercise involving external weight/resistance, use the highest level of weight/resistance you can lift for the designated number of repetitions with perfect form. In exercises involving no external resistance (close-grip push-up), simply perform the designated number of repetitions. Between sets, rest as long as necessary to perform the next set at the same level of performance, but no longer. When you see "A1" and "A2" or "B1" and "B2," etc., you should alternate between those two exercises. This phase includes Moving Day—your program-ending five-movement strength and power test.

PHASE 4 ENERGY WORKOUT RECOMMENDATIONS

Following are energy workout recommendations for Phase 4. Separate recommendations are provided for each of the three somatotypes discussed in Chapter 3.

Ectomorphs

TUESDAY AND THURSDAY. Technique practice (see page 24 for a sample technique practice session) with 30 percent of one-rep max, then 20 minutes of low-intensity cardio (at 60 to 70 percent of max heart rate).

Mesomorphs

IMMEDIATELY FOLLOWING EACH STRENGTH-TRAINING SESSION. Ten minutes of low-intensity cardio (cycling, running, etc., at 60 to 70 percent of max heart rate).

TUESDAY. Twenty minutes (excluding warm-up and cooldown) of high-intensity interval training on a 30-seconds work/60-seconds rest cycle on the elliptical trainer, bicycle, rower, or running.

THURSDAY. Technique practice (see page 24 for a sample technique practice session) with 30 percent of one-rep max, then 20 minutes of low-intensity cardio (at 60 to 70 percent of max heart rate).

Endomorphs

IMMEDIATELY FOLLOWING EACH STRENGTH-TRAINING SESSION. Ten minutes of low-intensity cardio (at 60 to 70 percent of max heart rate).

SATURDAY. Replace low-intensity postlifting cardio with 10 minutes of high-intensity interval training on a 30-seconds work/60-seconds rest cycle on the elliptical trainer, bicycle, rower, or running.

TUESDAY. Twenty minutes (excluding warm-up and cooldown) of high-intensity interval training on a 30-seconds work/60-seconds rest cycle on the elliptical trainer, bicycle, rower, or running.

THURSDAY. Technique practice (see page 24 for a sample technique practice session) with 30 percent of one-rep max, then 20 minutes of low-intensity cardio (at 60 to 70 percent of max heart rate).

MOVING DAY

All you have to do on Moving Day is repeat the pretesting protocol described in Phase 1, pages 77–80. Begin by weighing yourself as soon as you get out of bed. When you go to the gym, do a complete mobility warm-up, and then proceed through all five performance tests, including movement-specific warm-ups. Record your results in the table on the next page, to the right of your pretesting results. Try to have "after" photos taken later the same day, if possible.

PRETESTING AND MOVING DAY RESULTS

	PRETESTING	MOVING DAY
BODY WEIGHT		
BROAD JUMP		
BENCH PRESS		
BOX SQUAT		
DEADLIFT		
THREE-REP MAX CHIN-UP		

NOW WHAT?

Congratulations! You've completed the Maximum Strength Program, and you are stronger and fitter than you have ever been—or at least a hell of a lot stronger and fitter than you were 16 weeks ago. Now what? Take a well-earned day off, treat yourself to a cheat meal, and then get your ass back in the gym!

Yeah, but then what? Don't worry. Just flip ahead to Chapter 12 for some guidelines that will help you keep getting stronger and fitter for years to come. You didn't really think I was going to leave you hanging after Moving Day, did you?

CHAPTER 10

NUTRITION FOR MAXIMUM STRENGTH

We all know what a healthy diet is. A healthy diet is based on natural whole foods instead of processed foods, contains a balance of food types, and provides just enough total calories to sustain a healthy body weight. These are the eating habits that every legitimate nutrition expert recommends. However, I don't believe the standard healthy diet is quite adequate for individuals like us, who push our bodies' performance limits with physical training. Hard training places unusual stress on the body, and special nutritional measures are required to fully absorb and adapt to such stress, so that the stress builds the body up instead of breaking it down. An abundance of scientific research has shown that athletes perform better when they incorporate advanced nutrition practices that go beyond the standard recommendations.

One of my good friends and most esteemed colleagues is John Berardi, PhD, who is a leading expert on sports nutrition. (If his name sounds familiar, it's because he wrote the foreword to this book!) A few years ago, John created a comprehensive nutrition program for athletes and fitness enthusiasts called Precision Nutrition. I believe this program represents the perfect hybrid of simple, old-fashioned eating guidelines as described above *plus* a more cutting-edge, science-based set of guidelines based on the special nutritional needs of athletes.

The essence of the Precision Nutrition Program is a set of 10 eating habits. I recommend that you follow these guidelines while undertaking the Maximum Strength Program.

HABIT 1: EAT EVERY TWO OR THREE HOURS

Eating frequently is proven to elevate the body's metabolism and limit fat storage. If you eat, say, 3,000 calories in one day and distribute these calories among six separate eating occasions, your body will actually burn more of these calories to produce body heat than it will if you consume 3,000 calories in just two or three meals.

Another benefit of distributing your daily calories among a larger number of meals is that you consume fewer calories at each sitting. When you eat more calories than necessary to satisfy your body's immediate energy needs, many of the excess calories are stored as body fat. The larger your meals are, the more excess calories there will be, and the more fat you'll store. When you eat smaller meals more frequently, you are more likely to consume just enough calories at each sitting to meet your body's immediate energy needs, so fewer calories are stored as body fat. Here's a sensible eating schedule to follow:

7:00 A.M. — BREAKFAST

10:00 A.M. — MID-MORNING MEAL

12:00 P.M. — LUNCH

3:00 P.M. — MID-AFTERNOON MEAL

6:00 P.M. — DINNER

9:00 P.M. — PRE-BED MEAL

When you toss in a pre/during/post-training shake, you're actually looking at seven meals per day. Trust me: It's easier than it might sound!

HABIT 2: EAT A COMPLETE, LEAN PROTEIN ON EACH EATING OCCASION

Eating protein on each eating occasion is important for three reasons. First, it helps you achieve a high overall level of protein consumption, which is essential to maximize the muscle growth and strength gains resulting from your training sessions. Research has shown that increasing protein intake from normal levels (0.5–0.6 grams per pound of body weight daily) up to 0.7–0.8 grams per pound of body weight daily maximizes the muscle growth resulting from resistance exercise. However, most high-level body-builders and strength athletes (myself included) consume at least 1 gram of protein per pound of body weight daily. In this case, as in so many others, I think it's best to emulate what those with the biggest, strongest muscles do instead of what the laboratory results suggest.

Protein is also the most thermogenic macronutrient; that is, the body has to burn more calories to digest, absorb, and metabolize proteins than it does with either carbohydrates or fats. Consequently, a high-protein diet produces a higher metabolic rate and less fat storage than a moderate- to low-protein diet.

Finally, protein is generally believed to be the most filling of the three macronutrients. Thus, if you maintain a high-protein diet, you are less likely to overeat because of hunger.

The words *complete* and *lean* in the formulation of Habit 2 are significant. Not all proteins are complete, and not all proteins are lean. Proteins from plant sources are incomplete (i.e., they lack one or more essential amino acids), while those from animal sources are complete. So you should consume protein from an animal source on each eating occasion. But not all animal proteins are lean, that is, low-fat. Full-fat dairy foods and fatty meats are high in fat. Lean sources of animal protein include lean cuts of beef and pork; low-fat and nonfat dairy products; skinless poultry; fish; and powdered protein drink mixes.

If you are a lacto-ovo vegetarian, rely on nonfat and low-fat dairy foods, egg whites and the occasional whole egg, and milk protein supplements for most of your daily protein. If you're a vegan, don't expect to be able to build muscle and strength as quickly as you could if you included animal foods in your diet. Research proves that you can't.

HABIT 3: EAT VEGETABLES ON EACH EATING OCCASION

Vegetables are a rich source of lasting carbohydrate energy, vitamins and minerals, fiber, and antioxidants. Eating a vegetable-rich diet is proven to provide wide-ranging disease-prevention benefits. The U.S. Department of Agriculture recommends that men eat five servings of vegetables daily for optimal health. The only way you're likely to hit this target consistently is by getting in the habit of eating some type of vegetable at each sitting throughout the day.

Five servings a day sounds burdensome, but a serving is not large. A serving is defined as one-half cup of cooked vegetables or one cup of raw vegetables or salad. You can do that. In fact, if you ever find that it's not practical to consume vegetables in a particular meal or snack (how many convenient vegetable snacks can you name?), you can still easily meet your daily quota by doubling up at another meal.

For example, if you have a large two-cup salad as part of your lunch, a smoothie with eight ounces of orange juice and one cup of strawberries, and then four or five steamed asparagus spears with your dinner, you've just had *six* servings of fruits and vegetables in one day.

HABIT 4: EAT VEGGIES AND FRUITS WITH ANY MEAL, OTHER "CARBS" ONLY AFTER EXERCISE

As you probably know, carbohydrate-containing foods are classified by a tool called the *glycemic index.* High-glycemic carbs are absorbed quickly and provide a quick rush of energy that does not last long and often gives way to a subsequent feeling of lethargy (called *rebound hypoglycemia*). Low-glycemic carbs are absorbed more slowly and provide sustained energy. Higher-glycemic carbohydrate sources such as bread and pasta do a nice job of replenishing muscle fuel stores after exercise, but at other times their heavy carbohydrate load results in too much fat storage, because carbs that are not needed for immediate energy or glycogen stores are converted to fat and sent to the body's adipose tissues (which store fat in the body's midsection).

All vegetables and most fruits have a low glycemic index, so that the carbs they contain are less likely to be converted to stored fat. Some fruits are high-glycemic, but they contain fewer total carbohydrates than high-glycemic grain-based foods and sweets, so they still result in minimal fat storage, if any. Thus, fruits and vegetables are better sources of "anytime energy."

Note that, generally, your overall level of carbohydrate intake should vary with your training workload, since carbohydrate is your primary energy source for training. If the Maximum Strength Program represents a significant increase in your training workload and/or you find it difficult to maintain lean body mass during the early weeks of the program, you may need to increase your intake of healthy carbohydrates (vegetables, fruits, and whole grains)—so you can be a little less strict in following this particular habit. But most guys will get the best results by following Habit 4 to the letter.

HABIT 5: EAT HEALTHY FATS DAILY

There are three basic categories of fats: saturated, monounsaturated, and polyunsaturated. For optimal health you need to consume a balance of these three fat types. Most Americans consume too many saturated fats, too few monounsaturated fats, and the wrong kind of polyunsaturated fats. High levels of saturated fat consumption are closely associated with weight gain, obesity, and heart disease.

The ratio of unsaturated to saturated fats in the typical American diet is roughly 1:2. The ideal ratio is just the reverse, 2:1 (that is, twice as many unsaturated fats as saturated fats). The largest amounts of saturated fats are found, as you already know, in fatty cuts of meat, whole-milk dairy products, fried foods, and baked goods made with certain oils. You can easily and drastically reduce your saturated-fat consumption by limiting your consumption of these foods. Switch from fatty meats to lean meats, strictly limit the potato chips and french fries, and switch from whole-milk dairy foods to low-fat and nonfat dairy foods.

I'm sure you also know already that even worse than saturated fat, which is healthy in modest amounts, is trans fat, an artificial fat that is unhealthy in any amount. Trans fats are created when food chemists add hydrogen atoms to unsaturated fats to make them more saturated and, in turn, increase their melting point and make them better for baking and prolong their shelf life. Fortunately, the U.S. Food and Drug Administration now requires that trans fat content be listed on food package labels, so it's easier to eat around this most unhealthy type of fat. High levels of trans fat consumption have been shown to increase heart disease risk even more than high levels of saturated-fat consumption. Meanwhile, both polyunsaturated and monounsaturated fats lower total cholesterol and LDL (the bad cholesterol). *If you see trans fat on a product label, simply don't buy it.*

Good sources of polyunsaturated fats are fish, walnuts, and safflower oil. The most important polyunsaturated fats of all are the omega-3 fatty acids. The omega-3 fatty acids DHA and EPA are essential fatty acids (EFA); that is, they cannot be synthesized in the body, so they must be obtained in adequate amounts in the diet. This is easier said than done, as omega-3 fatty acids are destroyed when the oils that contain them are processed or heated, and most of the omega-3 sources in the modern diet are processed and/or heated. Many experts believe that omega-3 deficiency is one of the most widespread nutrient deficiencies in our society—and that's a sentiment I share from years of reviewing new clients' diets.

Omega-3s create healthier cell membranes. In addition, they are important precursors to anti-inflammatory components of the immune system. Omega-3 supplementation has been shown to improve cardiovascular health, sympathetic nervous system function, immune function, skin health, and a host of other health parameters. The best sources of omega-3 fatty acids are identical to the best sources of polyunsaturated fats in general: fatty types of fish (salmon, halibut, etc.), flax seeds, and walnuts. Unfortunately, there aren't many other foods that contain high levels of omega-3s. For this reason, I recommend that everyone take a daily fish oil supplement (see page 191).

There's another class of essential fats, called the omega-6 class, that you have probably also heard about. Omega-6 fatty acids are found abundantly in grains, eggs, and poultry. The typical American diet is not deficient in omega-6 fats, so you don't need to make any special effort to add them to your diet as you do with omega-3s.

Last but not least are the monounsaturated fats. Good sources of these healthier fats include olive oil, almonds, cashews, and natural peanut butter.

HABIT 6: DON'T DRINK BEVERAGES WITH MORE THAN ZERO CALORIES

One of the easiest ways to trim a surprising number of calories from your daily intake is to make a few key beverage substitutions. America has become a beverage-crazy society in the past quarter century, and this trend has had a significant impact on our bodies. The sheer variety of beverages available in stores has exploded, and serving sizes have also increased substantially. Currently, one in five calories in the average American's diet comes from beverages.

By replacing high-calorie beverages with zero-calorie beverages (preferably plain water), you can improve your body composition significantly without making any other changes in your diet. This strategy was demonstrated by a study done at Children's Hospital in Boston. Researchers there invited 103 teenagers to pick noncaloric drinks they liked and then delivered a supply of those drinks to their home refrigerators. Apparently, the kids actually drank the stuff, because consumption of sugar-sweetened beverages tumbled by 82 percent over six months. The subjects also lost one pound of body weight per month, on average, in the study period.

If you're serious about getting leaner and healthier, the only liquids you should regularly consume are water, green tea (a rich source of antioxidants with virtually no calories), and protein shakes.

HABIT 7: EAT WHOLE FOODS INSTEAD OF SUPPLEMENTS WHENEVER POSSIBLE

Your body was designed to absorb and metabolize natural, unprocessed foods, including fresh fruits and vegetables, seafood, and lean meats. Optimal health and performance are possible only if your diet is based on these foods. Nutritional supplements should have only a small place in your diet.

Some nutrition experts believe that nutritional supplements should be avoided altogether. My view is that this extreme position is not quite realistic, especially for men who push their bodies hard in the gym. If you're gunning for maximal strength, you need to consume fairly large amounts of protein frequently. Frankly, you can eat only so much meat. So there's nothing wrong with snacking on protein shakes and bars and chugging down high-protein posttraining drinks on the way home from the gym.

Believe it or not, research has actually shown that a pretraining shake containing protein (and carbs, ideally) improves long-term muscle mass gains more than a post-training shake alone. Unless you want to eat half a chicken breast immediately before you train and the other half immediately after you train, a good protein powder is your best bet. I recommend Biotest Surge as a pre/during/post-training protein source; you can find this and other protein powders online or at health food stores.

There are a handful of other nutritional supplements that are acceptable and even beneficial. Creatine supplements are proven to increase strength beyond the level that creatine-containing foods can. Fish oil supplements, as mentioned above, make it much easier to get the amount of omega-3 fatty acids that is needed for optimal health. I'll say more about each of these types of nutritional supplements later in the chapter.

HABIT 8: PLAN AHEAD AND PREPARE MEALS AND SNACKS IN ADVANCE

It's one thing to know what you ought to eat and when. It's another to actually eat what you should eat when you should eat it. Eating by the rules on a consistent basis requires a consistent effort to plan and prepare ahead of time so that you don't get stuck with the fast-food drive-through as your only option to cure a raging hunger. You should put the same degree of planning and preparation into your eating as you put into your training. You always know where and when you will do tomorrow's training session, and what sort of training you will do. Similarly, you should also know where and when you will eat tomorrow's meals, and more or less of what these meals will consist. And if any of these meals requires shopping and preparation, it's important that you take care of these things ahead of time.

There are a few simple measures you can take to ensure you always have the right foods available at the right times. One is to identify restaurants that serve healthy meals near where you'll be. If you are planning tomorrow's meals, and you know that you will be away from home for at least one of them and you are unable to take something with you, simply choose a restaurant from your list that you know you will be able to access for this meal, and order wisely.

Another measure you can take is to make sure your kitchen is always well stocked with lean protein sources, fresh vegetables, and other healthy foods. Pick one day of the week to do your food shopping for the following week, and err on the side of buying more than enough to get you through the next seven days, so you never run out of wholesome options and wind up calling the pizza delivery guy to bail you out. One strategy I've employed with great success is to cook in bulk on the weekends and freeze whatever I don't plan to use immediately. When things are hectic during the week, I can just defrost and chow down instead of having to cook an entire meal from scratch.

Stashing healthy snacks in your car and at work makes it easy to take care of your mid-morning and mid-afternoon needs. Options for the car and office include fruits, mixed nuts, low-carb beef jerky, protein powder, and protein bars (in a pinch).

Finally, I recommend that you build a repertoire of dinners and other menus that you can prepare at home. If you like to cook, this is easily done; you just have to find recipes that include lean protein, vegetables, variety, and no high-glycemic carbs (except after exercise). If you don't like to cook, you need to find recipes that meet these requirements and are very quick and easy to throw together. A great source of such recipes is the *Gourmet Nutrition* booklet that comes with Dr. Berardi's Precision Nutrition kit. Visit www.precisionnutrition.com to order it. Another good source is *Power Eating* by Susan Kleiner, PhD.

HABIT 9: EAT AS WIDE A VARIETY OF FOODS AS POSSIBLE

Different foods offer different nutrition profiles. No food provides every nutrient your body needs, and many natural foods provide nutrients that few or no other foods provide. This is especially true of plant foods, which contain dozens of useful *phytonutrients* (nonessential but highly beneficial plant nutrients, many of which function as antioxidants) that help the body in many ways. So the best way to ensure that your body gets enough of each nutrient is to consistently eat a wide variety of foods.

I'm not talking about merely hitting all of the basic food groups each day. I'm talking about getting as much variety as possible *within* each food group. Your animal protein should not always come from beef. Romaine lettuce should not be your only green vegetable. You get the idea.

The greatest potential source of variety in your diet comes from vegetables. Each type of vegetable has a nutrition profile that's a little different from that of any other. By mixing up the vegetables in your diet, you will supply your body with the greatest balance of healthful plant nutrients. The five categories are dark green, orange, legumes, starchy vegetables, and other vegetables. The table on page 186 lists examples of each.

Make an effort to consistently include vegetables from all five categories in your diet.

DARK GREEN	ORANGE	LEGUMES	STARCHY	OTHER
BOK CHOY	ACORN SQUASH	BLACK BEANS	CORN	ARTICHOKES
BROCCOLI	BUTTERNUT	BLACK-EYED PEAS	GREEN PEAS	ASPARAGUS
COLLARD	SQUASH	GARBANZO BEANS (CHICKPEAS)	POTATOES	BEETS
GREENS	CARROTS	KIDNEY BEANS		BRUSSELS SPROUTS
DARK GREEN	PUMPKIN	LENTILS		CABBAGE
LEAFY LETTUCE	SWEET POTATOES	LIMA BEANS		CAULIFLOWER
KALE		NAVY BEANS		CUCUMBERS
MUSTARD		PINTO BEANS		EGGPLANT
GREENS		SOYBEANS		GREEN BEANS
ROMAINE LETTUCE		SPLIT PEAS		OKRA
SPINACH		WHITE BEANS		ONIONS
TURNIP GREENS				SWEET PEPPERS
WATERCRESS				TOMATOES
				VEGETABLE JUICE
				ZUCCHINI

HABIT 10: DON'T "BREAK THE RULES" MORE THAN 10 PERCENT OF THE TIME

On the Precision Nutrition plan you will eat 6 times a day on average, or 42 times a week. In order to enjoy the full benefits of this system, you must break the rules no more than 10 percent of the time, or roughly 4 times a week. That's not much, so you should try to obey the rules every time you eat. When you do break a rule, consider it water under the bridge; don't have a guilt fit. Just move on and eat right next time, and the next time, and the next time.

THE CALORIE QUESTION

Most eating plans start by telling you how much you should eat and then tell you what (and possibly when) to eat. Precision Nutrition is different. In this system you may eat as much as you feel like eating. Why? Because if you follow the 10 Precision Nutrition habits, train consistently, and focus on performance as I've emphasized, you simply won't be able to eat more calories than your body needs to fuel and build your muscles.

Counting calories is totally unnecessary; I never have my clients do so. All you have to do is eat enough to feel comfortably satisfied at each meal. Over time, you learn to eat the right amount instinctively. The quality of your nutrition, the frequency of your feedings, and your hard work in the gym will combine to ensure that there will be no "extra" calories left over for fat storage after your muscles' needs have been met. Trust me.

A SAMPLE DAY OF PRECISION NUTRITION

Exactly how you put the Precision Nutrition principles into practice depends on when you train. The reason is that non-fruit-and-vegetable carbs are to be consumed only during the first two hours after training (and at breakfast, in those who tend to tolerate carbs well). Here are sample one-day eating plans for those who train in the morning (before work) and for those who train in the late afternoon or evening (after work).

MORNING TRAINING MEAL PLAN

TRAINING PRE/DURING/POST.	Biotest Surge shake (or comparable shake; never train on an empty stomach!).*
BREAKFAST.	¾ cup oats (dry measure) with two scoops low-carb chocolate whey protein powder (stirred in), one apple (or other fruit).
MID-MORNING MEAL.	Protein bar with one orange (or other fruit).
LUNCH.	Grilled chicken spinach salad with fresh veggies, olive oil and vinegar for dressing, fish oil soft gels (half of daily dosage).
MID-AFTERNOON MEAL.	One scoop low-carb protein powder mixed in water and ¼ cup almond/walnut mixture.
DINNER.	Lean red meat with steamed vegetables.
PRE-BED MEAL.	Smoothie with one scoop low-carb vanilla protein powder, ½ cup blueberries (or other berries), ice, and ½ cup cottage cheese; one tablespoon natural peanut butter (eaten separately); fish oil soft gels (half of daily dosage).

*NOTE: Those looking to get leaner should use half the recommended dose of protein powder and add one scoop of low-carb protein powder instead.

EVENING TRAINING MEAL PLAN

BREAKFAST.	Omelet with eggs (two or three) plus one or two additional egg whites with veggies (chopped onions, tomatoes, spinach, and diced tomatoes), fish oil soft gels (half of daily dosage).
MID-MORNING MEAL.	One scoop low-carb protein powder mixed in water and ¼ cup almonds or other nuts; fish oil soft gels.
LUNCH.	Spinach salad with additional veggies and grilled chicken and olive oil and vinegar for dressing, fish oil soft gels (half of daily dosage).
MID-AFTERNOON MEAL.	1 cup low-fat cottage cheese with ¼ cup raspberries, ¼ cup walnuts (or other fruit or nuts).
TRAINING PRE/DURING/POST.	Biotest Surge shake.*
DINNER.	Grilled chicken; sweet potato; green beans.
EVENING SNACK.	Smoothie with one scoop low-carb vanilla protein powder, ½ cup blueberries, ice, and ½ cup cottage cheese; one pear (or other fruit).

SUPPLEMENTS WORTH CONSIDERING

So much money is spent on the marketing and advertising of nutritional supplements that it's difficult to avoid being brainwashed. The underlying message of these communications is that you cannot maximize your health and athletic performance without nutritional supplements. The reality is that only a very small number of supplements are scientifically proven to enhance the benefits of resistance exercise, and their effect is modest.

In other words, in the pursuit of maximal strength, supplements are optional. The four primary nutritional supplements that I consider worth a try for virtually everyone are creatine, fish oil, protein blends, and vegetable supplements.

Creatine

Creatine phosphate occurs naturally in the body and is one of the most important sources of energy for high-intensity (anaerobic) muscle contractions. Creatine phosphate is able to provide energy so rapidly that it is the muscles' primary energy source for maximum-intensity efforts such as heavy weightlifting and sprinting. The muscles store it in extremely small amounts, though, so it lasts no longer than 15 seconds during maximum-intensity muscle work.

A tiny percentage of our creatine phosphate stores is synthesized in the body. The rest comes ready-made in protein-rich foods, including fish and beef. But even these foods contain only small amounts of creatine phosphate. That's why scientists in the 1990s began to look at creatine supplementation as a potential means to enhance high-intensity muscle performance (strength, speed, and power) by increasing the availability of this particular energy source in the muscles. They quickly found that various creatine phosphate precursors, including creatine monohydrate, are readily converted to creatine phosphate in the body and, when taken supplementally, increase creatine phosphate stores in the muscles far beyond the levels that can be achieved by diet alone.

As few as five days of creatine monohydrate supplementation increase creatine phosphate levels in the body by 10 to 40 percent. Dozens of research studies have shown that these increases translate directly into faster muscle development and strength building. However, some people find that creatine has little effect. Scientists refer to these individuals as "nonresponders." And even among the majority of individuals who do respond to creatine supplementation, some benefit more than others, so if you're interested in trying it, you'll just have to see what it does for you.

I recommend that you take three to five grams per day. You can mix the powder into any drink, but most lifters prefer to just include it with their pre/during/posttraining shake. On off days, simply stir it into your green tea. Do not fall for the hype that says that you need a special creatine delivery system full of carbs and a thousand other ingredients. Plain old powdered creatine is very affordable and is all you need to get the job done. You do not need to worry about beginning the supplementation process with a "loading phase," either; simply taking a small dosage over the course of three to four weeks will get you the same results without any of the minor gastrointestinal problems (stomach bloating and gas) that come with loading.

There has been some public concern about side effects associated with creatine supplementation, including muscle cramping and altered liver and kidney function. However, formal scientific studies have found no evidence of any side effects, except muscle weight gain, and recent comprehensive reviews of the literature have concluded that even long-term creatine supplementation is safe. If you have questions, ask your doctor.

Fish Oil

The American Heart Association recommends that we eat fish at least twice a week to nourish our bodies with healthy fat. But eating fish twice a week or even daily doesn't provide enough of the essential fatty acids EPA and DHA to meet the body's needs. A good rule of thumb is to aim for a combined 3,000 milligrams of EPA and DHA per day. The majority of products out on the market provide 180 milligrams EPA and 120 milligrams DHA per soft gel. Thus, you need 10 soft gels per day to reach your "quota." While it sounds like a ton, it amounts to only a few teaspoons of oil. Fortunately, some companies have created more concentrated versions to make our lives easier. Biotest's Flameout, for instance, provides the necessary daily total in only four soft gels. Carlson also makes a quality liquid fish oil that you can use to get your allotted dose quite easily. It's fairly easy these days to find fish oil, whether it's at the corner drugstore or at your local health food store.

Regardless of the form you choose, I recommend that you take a fish oil supplement every day. Fish oil can help prevent arthritis, heart disease, psychological disorders, gastrointestinal problems, eye issues, and dozens of other maladies that relate to systemic inflammation. Think of it as giving your body the right raw materials with which to build cell membranes.

Protein Blends

As I mentioned above, most successful strength and power athletes (and bodybuilders) consume at least 1 gram of protein per pound of body weight. It is difficult to achieve this level of protein consumption in a calorically efficient way with whole-food protein sources alone. For example, to get 25 grams of protein from lean ground beef, you have to consume roughly 210 total calories. Meanwhile, you need to eat 250 calories of non-fat yogurt to get 25 grams of protein. To get the same amount of protein from a whey protein powder, though, you have to consume only 120 calories. (Although you don't need to count calories on the Precision Nutrition plan, half the reason you don't have to count calories is that it's based on calorically efficient foods.) Protein supplements also afford us more convenience when we're on the go, and around exercise times, when the last thing we want to do is eat solid food. For these two reasons, I believe that including a powdered-protein drink mix in your daily nutrition regimen is a good idea.

The most popular type of protein supplement is whey. Whey protein is one of two main proteins in milk (the other is casein). It is one of the highest-quality proteins in nature, as it contains all 20 amino acids and high levels of the specific amino acids that are known to be most important for muscle performance and growth (leucine, isoleucine, valine, and glutamine, in particular). Whey protein is also absorbed and metabolized very quickly compared to other proteins. For this reason, it's a great choice around training times, when you want protein to go to work quickly.

Personally, I prefer protein supplements that combine fast-acting whey protein with slower-acting proteins such as casein. While no protein matches the capacity of whey to increase muscle protein synthesis around a training session, casein actually does a better job of reducing muscle protein breakdown (which is normally elevated after training). Thus, a supplement that combines whey and casein has a more positive effect on net muscle protein balance. If you're using these supplements during the day as a meal replacement product, opt for low-carb versions and combine them with solid foods (e.g., nuts, fruit).

Other research has shown that protein supplementation is most effective when the supplement is consumed either immediately before or immediately after training. The objective is to make amino acids readily available when the muscles begin their recovery and adaptive response to training in the hours following a training session.

The typical whey protein supplement provides approximately 20 to 25 grams of protein per serving, which is plenty. Research has shown that combining whey protein consumption with carbohydrate consumption around training times enhances the muscle-building effects of whey protein supplementation. It does so by stimulating a greater release of insulin, which delivers amino acids into the muscle cells and initiates muscle protein synthesis. The easiest way to get the combination of protein and carbs you need to maximize muscle protein synthesis after training sessions is to consume a post-training recovery drink such as Surge by Biotest (www.biotest.net) instead of a pure protein supplement.

Vegetable Supplements

If you are able to consistently eat five or more servings of vegetables daily, good for you. But only a quarter of American adults manage to consume even three servings of vegetables daily. Vegetable-based nutrition supplements can help fill the gap. You can purchase capsules and powders made of extracts from a large variety of vegetables, fruits, and herbs.

I'm not saying that vegetable supplements represent an equivalent alternative to whole vegetables, but they do deliver a lot of nutrition and are better than skimping on veggies altogether. You can find them at many health food stores.

SUPPLEMENTS TO AVOID

The vast majority of nutritional supplements that are sold under muscle-building (and fat-burning) claims are scientifically proven to have no effect on muscle growth or strength gains. In other words, if you buy them, you're a sucker. My list of the top supplements to avoid wasting your money on includes arginine, chromium picolinate, DHEA, HMB, and ribose.

Arginine

Several years ago, supplements that are purported to elevate nitric oxide (NO) production in the body became popular among men seeking muscle growth and strength gains. Blood vessels produce nitric oxide, which helps them dilate to increase blood flow. With increased blood flow comes increased oxygen and nutrient delivery to the muscles and fuller, more "pumped"-looking muscles. The amino acid arginine is one of the main substrates for NO synthesis and is the main ingredient in most of the many NO-boosting supplements on the market. However, natural arginine levels far exceed anything you can take in pill form (without GI distress) to stimulate NO production.

The majority of these supplements are marketed with claims that they increase muscle size and strength. However, there is absolutely no scientific basis for these claims. In fact, arginine supplementation has been shown to mute the growth hormone response to resistance training, so it can actually *limit* mass and strength gains than to augment them.

Chromium Picolinate

An essential trace mineral (i.e., a mineral humans need in very small amounts), chromium is naturally present in foods such as beef, eggs, and spinach. It is also an ingredient in many diet products because chromium is known to assist naturally in the metabolism of carbs and fats, as well as in blood sugar regulation. Many bodybuilders take chromium supplements—usually in the form of chromium picolinate—in the belief that it helps them burn fat and improve their body composition.

[For the life of me I can't figure out why anyone takes supplemental chromium picolinate. Study after study has found that it is completely ineffective.] For example, one study from the University of Maryland compared the effects of daily chromium picolinate supplementation with a placebo during 12 weeks of resistance training. The study's authors concluded, "Chromium supplementation, in conjunction with a progressive, resistive exercise training program, does not promote a significant increase in strength and lean body mass, or a significant decrease in percent body fat."

Dehydroepiandrosterone

Dehydroepiandrosterone (DHEA) is a relatively weak steroid hormone similar to estrogen and testosterone. Synthetic DHEA is sold as a supplement under claims that it slows the aging process, including the muscle and strength declines that are part of aging, and protects against a variety of diseases and ailments, including heart disease and Alzheimer's disease.

The original rationale for DHEA supplementation was the fact that DHEA levels naturally peak at age 25 and decline thereafter, roughly in parallel with testosterone levels in men. It was thought that supplementation might slow and to some degree reverse this hormonal decline and any aging processes that might be connected to it. Early studies with rodents looked promising, but the trouble is that rodents produce very little DHEA, so the results did not translate. Recent human studies, including a large two-year study at the Mayo Clinic, have found that DHEA supplementation fails to increase testosterone levels or muscle size and strength gains resulting from resistance exercise.

Beta-hydroxy beta-methylbutyrate

Beta-hydroxy beta-methylbutyrate (HMB) is a metabolite of the essential amino acid leucine. HMB became popular as a muscle- and strength-building supplement in the 1990s because of speculation that it might limit muscle protein degradation following resistance exercise and enhance positive nitrogen balance. The effects of HMB on muscle and strength gains resulting from resistance training have since been investigated in numerous studies. Some have shown that it is effective, while others have shown that it is not.

The majority of studies showing benefits have been poorly designed. A majority of the well-designed studies have shown no benefit. Also, most studies showing beneficial effects of HMB supplementation have involved beginning weightlifters, while most studies involving trained weightlifters have shown no benefit. While there may be a small benefit to HMB at very high dosages, looking at the total pool of research on HMB I can say with confidence that HMB supplementation is not worth the $50 to $60 per month it would cost you!

Ribose

Ribose is a sugar that the body produces through glucose metabolism and is in turn used to replenish adenosine triphosphate (ATP) stores in muscle cells. Therefore, it plays an important role in muscle energy production. Many bodybuilders and strength athletes use ribose supplements in the belief that these accelerate muscle recovery by increasing the rate of ATP synthesis after training.

However, studies have demonstrated unequivocally that ribose does not have this effect. For example, in a double-blind, randomized, placebo-controlled Belgian study, subjects performed an intensive regimen of lower-body strength exercises over a six-day period. Subjects who took a ribose supplement neither replenished ATP stores faster than placebo subjects nor outperformed them in strength tests.

There are literally hundreds of other supplements out there on which people willingly spend money, but from which they get little to no benefit. Covering them all would be beyond the scope of this book, but I hope by presenting these few examples I will save you some cash that could otherwise be spent on high-quality whole foods.

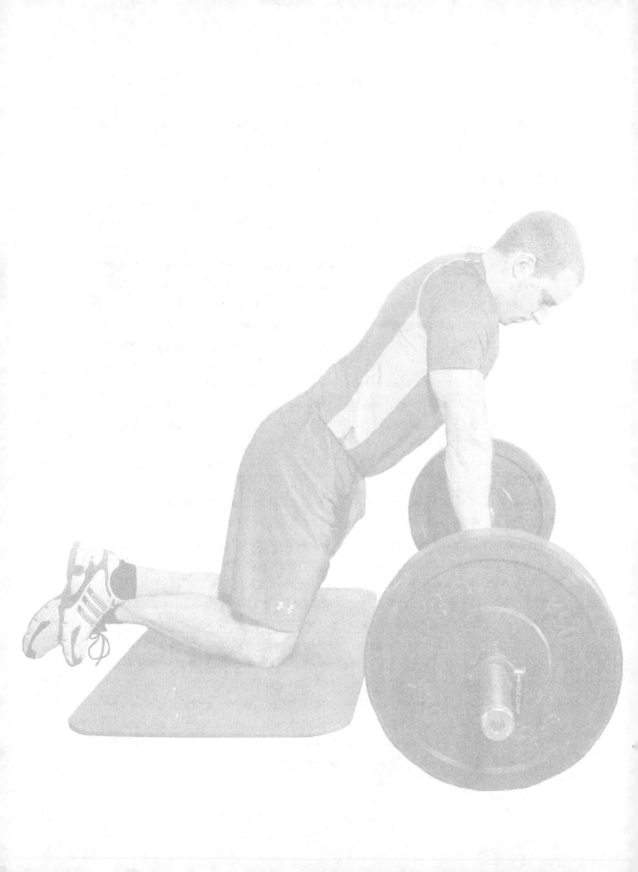

CHAPTER 11

THE MUSCLE BETWEEN YOUR EARS

Yogi Berra once said that half of baseball is 90 percent mental. Well, I believe that half of weightlifting is 90 percent mental, too. Whatever that means.

A lot of weightlifters take pride in having a dismissive attitude toward the mental aspect of resistance training. They feel that paying attention to the nuances of the mental side of pumping iron is a sign of mental weakness or softness. There's a funny contradiction inherent in this attitude. The notion that mental toughness enhances resistance-training performance, and that paying too much attention to one's thoughts and emotions saps mental toughness, is itself a way of recognizing the importance of the mind in relation to resistance-training performance. Besides being contradictory, this attitude is also just plain wrong. Without a doubt, mental toughness is a good thing, but just as surely, you cannot maximize your performance in the gym by simply trying to ignore your mind. You have to know how to harness its power.

Like it or not, your mind has tremendous influence over your muscles. You can't lift a pencil without it. For example, studies have shown that people are able to recruit more muscle fibers for a maximal voluntary muscle contraction when they are given verbal encouragement from others than when they are not. Other studies have shown that people can lift more weight when in competition with individuals of roughly equal strength than when competing only against themselves. Most competitive powerlifters are able to lift 10 percent more weight in competition than they can at any time in training. Certain types of music are scientifically proven to enhance strength, while others sap it. More than one study has found that people lift more weight when they are told they are lifting less than they really are, and that they lift less weight when they are told they are lifting more than they really are. And believe it or not, even the color of paint on the walls of a weightroom has been shown to affect strength performance.

There's just no getting around the fact that half of weightlifting is 90 percent mental. If you know how to use your mind skillfully, you will perform much better than you will if you vaguely try to be "tough." In this chapter, I will share with you some of my secrets to success in five areas related to the mental side of strength training: getting in the zone, what to think about during a lift, the importance of your training environment, dealing with setbacks, and knowing when to say when.

GETTING IN THE ZONE

Some mental and emotional states are more conducive to strength performance than others. The ideal state for most people is a focused state with few mental distractions and an eagerness for hard work. Your mind should not be cluttered with too many thoughts about the outside world.

Low motivation to train is probably the worst mental state to bring to the gym, but there's such a thing as being excessively amped, as well. Inexperienced lifters often assume that they are supposed to psych themselves up for lifts the way football players psych themselves up for games—knocking helmets and all that. These antics probably won't help you lift any more weight, but they might make you look like an ass to the other people who have to share the gym with you! None of the incredible lifters with whom I've trained has ever ripped down the door of the gym, screaming, "Let me at that bar!" They're motivated, no doubt, but they are all business in the way they put that motivation to use.

Here are some simple things you can do to put your mind in the right state for a productive training session.

Go Incommunicado

Turn off your cell phone well before you get to the gym to separate yourself from the outside world.

Cue Up Your Theme Music

If there's a particular kind of music that gets you motivated to exert yourself, play it on the drive over to the gym.

Ease into It

If you're coming to the gym straight from a hectic day at work, take a few moments to gather your thoughts before you throw yourself into the fire. Starting your training session with soft tissue and mobility work is very effective in this regard. It serves as an emotional transition period between your life outside the gym and the hard muscle work in which you're about to engage.

Fuel for Performance

Many weightlifters like to use pretraining nutritional supplements to prepare the mind and body for performance. The traditional choice is caffeine. A good caffeine jolt will stimulate your nervous system and elevate your mood. That's why its use is regulated by the International Olympic Committee and the National Collegiate Athletic Association (NCAA). But caffeine is just the tip of the iceberg in terms of pretraining supplementation these days. You've got guys using thiamine disulphide, tyrosine, dimethylaminoethanol (DMAE), gingko biloba, piracetam, citrulline malate, beta-alanine, and other unpronounceable compounds. Some guys feel they get great results from particular pretraining supplements while others do not. These days there are hundreds of nutritional supplements designed specifically to prepare body and mind for exercise. Research them thoroughly before choosing one to try (and don't feel obligated to choose any of them). Ultimately, whether any of these choices is right for you is something only you can determine.

Have a Plan

Having a plan in place for your training session before you even arrive at the gym makes it easier to focus on the task at hand. As I suggested above, experienced, high-level weightlifters take a businesslike approach to their training sessions. Knowing exactly what you will do in each session prior to starting it facilitates this approach by laying out in black and white precisely what sort of business is on the agenda. In the long term, you will get better results from your training if you show up at the gym each day with a businesslike attitude and a specific plan than you will if you arrive in a state of bug-eyed, frothing-mouthed madness to pump iron and with no plan at all.

The Maximum Strength Program takes care of your planning needs for you. Still, even after you "graduate" from this program, I urge you always to use detailed plans to guide your training.

WHAT TO THINK ABOUT DURING A LIFT

Your brain has various parts that are responsible for handling various functions. The part that has the primary responsibility for activating your muscles during a lift is the motor center. Other parts of your brain handle duties such as remembering past events from your day before you got to the gym, worrying about whether other guys in the gym are laughing at you for lifting such puny weights, and thinking about an important presentation you have to make at work tomorrow. At most times, several parts of the brain are active simultaneously, meaning that the brain is busily multitasking—even during activities such as weightlifting. But brain-imaging studies have shown that skilled athletes have a remarkable ability to quiet every part of the brain except for the motor center when they are training or competing. They basically stop thinking and shut down every irrelevant feeling and emotion, leaving only the brain's muscle "puppet master" in operation.

This is what you need to do when performing every repetition of every set in every session. You want to become what I call a "motor moron." Take your conscious thought processes completely out of the act. Don't think about work, or wonder what the bigger guys in the gym think of you, or try to steal a glance at the sexy gym bunny bending forward for a drink at the water fountain. Eliminate all distractions and focus all of your conscious attention on the lift itself. Use the detailed exercise descriptions provided in previous chapters to perform each repetition of the exercise with impeccable technique. Don't let your thoughts wander. There's plenty of time for that between sets.

The key to practicing this mental skill successfully is to focus your thoughts on the position and movement of your body. If you fill your mind with the sensation of tightening your core properly before executing a cable pull-through and recruiting every available muscle fiber that is capable of contributing to locking out your last repetition of a three-rep set of bench presses, there will be little or no room left in your skull for irrelevant thoughts.

Your goal is to make perfect technique virtually automatic on every exercise. The more precisely you are able to duplicate the most efficient movement patterns when you do any given exercise, the stronger you will become in that lift. When I look at videos of my performances at powerlifting meets, every deadlift I do is identical, and that's why the deadlift is my strength, so to speak. But when I look at my squat, my setup is a little different each time, and that's why I'm not as strong a squatter. I'm working on that.

Flaws in lifting technique are always specific in nature. Maybe you break with your knees instead of your hips when you initiate a squat, or you push too much through your forefeet instead of your heels when deadlifting. One of the most productive ways to focus your conscious attention on your body when performing any lift is to use proprioceptive cues to correct the biggest flaws in your technique. A proprioceptive cue is a word, phrase, or image that you think about while lifting in order to better control your technique. For example, if you tend to break the knees first when squatting, you can work to correct this flaw by concentrating on pushing your hips back, possibly to a target such as a box (as in box squats), and consciously tell yourself, "Sit back," on each rep. If you need to get better about keeping your weight back on your heels when deadlifting, you can wiggle your big toes or think about pushing your heels through the floor. Over time, I've actually become known for a "heel stomp" component of my deadlift that is completely unique to me; I don't teach it to any of my athletes, but it's worked to improve the precision of my deadlifting technique.

The more proficient you become in each exercise, the more you will be able to trust pure proprioception—the feel of your muscles and joints—to guide your execution. You will know the precise feeling of doing it right, and any deviation will feel wrong.

That said, no weightlifter can perfect his technique in any lift without the assistance of a coach or trainer. Not only do these professionals have knowledge of proper technique, but they can watch you in ways that you can never watch yourself and point out errors you would never notice, even if you are an expert on weightlifting technique yourself. So don't be too proud to seek out the help of a qualified weightlifting coach or a specialist in strength and conditioning at any point in your development, whether it's your very first day in the gym or your first day of training to qualify for your third Olympic team.

THE IMPORTANCE OF
YOUR TRAINING ENVIRONMENT

If you train alone in a pink-painted gym that plays elevator music on its sound system, you probably will not improve as quickly as you will if you train instead with good training partners in a white-painted gym that plays more up-tempo music on its sound system. In other words, your training environment is very important. Try to train at a gym that you like going to—where you feel comfortable, at home, and motivated to work hard.

For some guys, the ideal training environment is a "hard-core" lifters' gym with no mirrors on the walls, no machines, and few female members. Loud, angry, "my-mother-didn't-love-me" heavy metal is the music of choice. Rusty barbells and a lack of air-conditioning make the experience all the more enjoyable. For other guys, the ideal training environment is an upscale gym with pristine equipment, child care services, and a juice bar. There is no right or wrong choice for everyone; whatever works best for you is the right choice for you. Hard-core powerlifting gyms (my personal preference) are harder to find than the major fitness club franchises, but completely worth the effort, in my opinion. For assistance in locating powerlifting gyms in your area, log onto www.PowerliftingWatch.com and use the gym locator tool.

If possible, get involved with a training group of like-minded people who can push you a little more than you can push yourself. One way to find such people is to check out some of the various online weightlifting forums (www.T-Nation.com, www.JPFitness.com, www.EliteFTS.com) and submit a post letting others know that you're looking for a training partner in your area. The chances of actually meeting good training partners face-to-face are much greater at the hard-core powerlifting gyms you will find through the www.PowerliftingWatch.com gym locator than at the major health club franchises. And if all else fails, send me an e-mail (ec@ericcressey.com). I know maximum-strength seekers all across the country, so just let me know in your message where you are and that you're interested in meeting up with training partners, and I will do my best to put you in touch with likely candidates in your area.

If you can't find an existing group to join, recruit some buddies to create one. I can't overemphasize the difference that the right training group can make in terms of motivating you to train more consistently and with greater intensity. The year I lifted at South Side Gym in Stratford, Connecticut, was without a doubt the most productive training period of my career because I had to bust my ass just to avoid embarrassing myself. I went from being a big fish in a small pond at the University of Connecticut, where I could hold my own with all of the varsity athletes, to being the lightest member in South Side history. I was in there with guys who had benched 800 pounds, squatted 1,000 pounds, and done some other insane things. For the first three months, I just kept my mouth shut, helped load and unload plates, and tried to earn respect by lifting heavy stuff. I know that I made much more progress there than I would have made anywhere else because of the type of people who surrounded me. This is a mind-set that I've brought to my current training facility in Boston, and I've worked to foster this approach in my athletes and new training partners.

The ideal training partners are ones who are a little stronger than you are—at least in some lifts. Tennis legend Pete Sampras used to lose matches in the 18-and-under class when he could have won them in the 12-and-under class, and that's what made him the youngest-ever male singles champion at the U.S. Open in 1990 at the age of 19 years and 28 days, not to mention the owner of more Grand Slam singles titles (14) than any other man in history. Don't be afraid to start out as the weakest guy in a training group. Swallow your ego and allow yourself to be pulled along by your physical superiors. This approach will make you stronger in the long run.

DEALING WITH SETBACKS

There are three types of setbacks that you might face in training for maximum strength: poor training performances, low motivation, and injuries. There are good and bad ways of dealing with each of them. Let me explain the best ways.

Poor Training Performances

In any intense training program—and the Maximum Strength Program is certainly one of them—there are times when you will feel somewhat beaten down. Your muscles, carrying fatigue from recent hard training sessions, will feel hollowed-out and tender. Consequently, you will not be able to lift as much weight as you normally do. Your poor performance may affect your morale, causing you to lose focus and thus perform even more poorly.

While it is natural to want to get stronger in every lifting session, it is not realistic, and it's important to know that you can have some of your best sessions on those unavoidable days when you feel beaten down. I don't mean "best" in the sense that you lift more weight, because clearly that's just the opposite of what happens in such sessions. I mean "best" in the sense that you get the most out of them. If you refuse to lose morale and focus on your tough days and instead suffer gamely through your planned session (with slightly reduced loads, if necessary) despite lacking your usual strength, you will be rewarded with a greater training effect that allows you to lift more weight on your next good day.

Additionally, it's important to note that training stress fluctuates by design in the Maximum Strength Program. Consequently, there are bound to be times when you feel a bit beaten down, and times when you feel amped up and ready to move big weights. You'll begin to realize that the high and very-high-workload weeks will leave you a bit drained, while you feel rejuvenated at the end of the low-workload weeks—and that's the ideal time to display the fitness you've gained from the weeks that imposed all of that fatigue.

A substandard performance is just water under the bridge. People get so caught up in how much weight they're lifting that they forget about all of the benefits— endocrine, neuromuscular, cardiovascular, mental, and immune system—they can still get from a tough session where their performance is not the best. It's not how much weight you lift relative to your normal standards that counts. It's how hard you work. If you work equally hard on both your good days and your bad days, you will make more progress than you will if you throw yourself only into your best training sessions.

Low Motivation

The same principle applies to those days when you don't feel bad physically, but your motivation to train is low. You should never skip a session simply because you don't feel like working out. Don't even consider it an option. Regardless of where your head is, make sure your body does the same thing on your low-motivation days as it does on any other training day: It goes to the gym and it lifts hard!

At first, it might be difficult to overcome the temptation to take a day off, but the more times you resist your lazy instincts the easier it will become. And as you experience the rewards that come from maintaining perfect consistency in your training, overcoming low motivation will become even easier. I've missed only one planned training session in the last eight years, and that was because 35 inches of snow fell that day.

I wound up making up the session the next day. Consistency is what has made me successful, and it will do the same for you.

Injuries

Injuries are the worst kind of setback, because even the best mental attitude in the world won't enable you to train "normally" with certain injuries. While injuries—both acute and chronic—are certainly always a possibility with physical activity, the Maximum Strength Program is specifically designed to minimize injury risk while building strength. However, it cannot completely eliminate the possibility of injury.

I specialize in corrective exercise with athletes. These individuals are highly motivated to heal and return to normal training. They are willing to do whatever it takes to get back on the field, the court, the ice, or wherever it is they compete. And I am willing to do whatever it takes to help them—and that means getting as creative as I have to be to enable them to maintain (or even improve) fitness while working with physical therapists to correct the underlying cause of the injury and then resume training in a way that minimizes the risk of injury recurrence. Doctors often tell them what they *can't* do. I tell them what they *can* do.

I believe every injured exerciser should treat himself as an athlete, not a patient. There's always something you can do. Figure out what you can do and do it. And if you can't figure it out on your own, find a coach like me who can help you. It's worth the effort and the expense. If you're in pain, by all means, seek treatment from a sports orthopedist, but complement this treatment with aggressive efforts to train around your injury (that is, to continue exercising in ways you can do it pain-free).

Dealing with injuries is one area where it pays to be "mentally tough" in the old-school sense of this phrase. A recent study involving injured male soldiers found that those who scored higher on a test designed to assess traditionally masculine psychological traits (including unwillingness to complain about internal pain and suffering) tended to heal faster. The authors of the study speculated that men who are more reticent to communicate their suffering to others may also have a stronger belief in their ability to overcome suffering on their own, and that this belief is to some degree self-fulfilling.

Don't overinterpret this study. If you have a painful injury that needs medical treatment, by all means get treatment. But keep a positive attitude as well. Refuse to get discouraged. Believe in your power to heal and you will heal faster.

KNOWING WHEN TO SAY WHEN

There is such a thing as being *too* motivated to work out. When people become excessively focused on their goal of getting stronger, they sometimes push hard when their bodies are not in a fit state to absorb and benefit from heavy lifting. When your body is carrying an unusually high amount of fatigue from recent training, a heavy-lifting session will not stimulate positive muscle adaptations. It will only cause more fatigue to accumulate in your body, leading to *maladaptation*.

The temptation to push hard all the time stems from a tacit assumption that only heavy lifting increases strength. This is not the case. Other types of training, such as mobility and activation work, contribute indirectly to strength development as well. On days when your body cannot benefit from heavy lifting, it can still benefit from these other types of training. My feeling is that there's always something you can do to move toward your goals, even if you're too fatigued to lift heavy. It doesn't have to be all or nothing: doing your session as planned or skipping it completely. You can modify the session in a sensible way based on how you feel. On those days when I don't feel good, I'm not going to put 600 pounds on my back. The risks are too great and the potential rewards too small.

Another factor that contributes to strength building is deloading, or reducing your training workload temporarily to give your body a chance to fully absorb your recent hard training. Few people fully appreciate the benefits of deloading. I do my last heavy deadlift roughly one month before a meet. In the last week before the meet, I feel so strong and stir crazy it takes all the willpower I have not to bust down the door of the gym and do a heavy pull or two. But my approach pays off. In competition, it's not unusual to see lifters exceed their training "max" by as much as 10 percent thanks to deloading and the emotional stimuli associated with a competition.

The Maximum Strength Program includes a deloading week prior to Moving Day. When you get there, you'll see what I mean. You will feel like you could lift a truck, and who knows? You just might!

CHAPTER 12

MAXIMUM STRENGTH FOR LIFE

Congratulations! You've completed the Maximum Strength Program. Now you can cancel your gym membership and never train again for the rest of your life. You can also go back to eating 10 fast-food meals a week. Of course, you'll wind up looking like the Pilsbury Doughboy, getting dumped by your girlfriend, and living in your parents' basement. With that powerful image in mind, why not use the past 16 weeks as a foundation for a bigger, better, and *stronger* future?

For better or worse, maximum strength training and fueling your body for maximum strength are habits that you have to maintain consistently if you want to continue to enjoy their benefits and progress toward future goals. You could simply repeat the Maximum Strength Program over and over, exactly as it is presented in this book. At 16 weeks in length, it fits neatly into a year three times with 4 weeks left over for recovery, vacations, and alternate activities. But this pattern would start to feel stale after a while. One of the merits of the Maximum Strength Program is that it is more varied and progressive than the typical fitness routine. However, to keep things interesting and keep making gains over a period of years, you need more variation and progression than you will get by indefinitely repeating the Maximum Strength Program.

You'll get the best long-term results if your future training retains the core principles that are embedded in the Maximum Strength Program, and you fiddle with the details of your training in ways that allow you to build continually on past progress. The following 10 guidelines will help you strike this balance of consistency and variation and successfully pursue maximum strength for life.

STAY FOCUSED ON PERFORMANCE

The number one difference between the Maximum Strength Program and the programs you will find in most fitness books is that it is squarely focused on performance. What this means is that the program is specifically designed to enhance your body's core physical capabilities. Focusing on improving performance rather than on less tangible benefits such as changing your appearance is better because it is ultimately more fun and engaging and yields better all-around results.

I strongly recommend that you remain focused on performance in your future training. It takes many years of consistent, progressive training to reach one's lifetime limit of strength. If you want to get even stronger than you are now, make this goal the explicit objective of your future training and you will see improvement for a long time to come. My experience has been that staring at the scale and waiting anxiously to fill out that extra-large T-shirt is no way to set yourself up for long-term success. Chasing high-level performance on strength tasks will help you get bigger, if that's what you really want.

You can even switch over to new and different performance goals that are not strictly strength-related, if you so desire. Any performance goal is a good goal, as long as it's consistent with overall health. Aim to jump higher, run faster, win a lumberjack contest, or even tackle a triathlon, if it makes you happy!

CONTINUE TO SET
QUANTIFIABLE GOALS

Staying focused on performance and setting quantifiable goals go hand in hand. Performance is always measured with numbers. Aiming to increase your maximum lift in various strength movements is one of the most simple and straightforward performance goals you can set. The reason such goals are so important is that they tend to increase motivation and make the training process more linear and efficient. Goals such as wanting to look better and to stay in shape are too amorphous to provide the same level of motivation or the same selective pressure to use in deciding how to train most productively.

Except when you are enjoying a brief training break or deloading period, you should always work toward quantifiable goals. These goals may have short (weeks), intermediate (months), or long (a year or more) time spans, but at least one of them should be near enough to keep you focused and inspired in the gym. The 16-week goal horizon used in the Maximum Strength Program is a good standard to use when setting and pursuing future goals.

While performance goals are indispensable, they are not the only useful type of quantifiable goal to pursue. You may also set quantifiable health-related goals, such as achieving a certain body fat percentage or lowering your LDL cholesterol by a certain amount.

DON'T NEGLECT THE SMALL STUFF

If the Maximum Strength Program has taught you only one thing, I hope it has taught you the importance of making the health of your musculoskeletal system your very first priority in the gym. This is the true foundation for gains in strength. You are only as strong as your weakest link. Poor musculoskeletal health—in the form of lack of mobility, postural misalignment, and muscle strength imbalances—is the weak link for the vast majority of weightlifters.

In the Maximum Strength Program you attacked this weak link by warming up with mobility exercises, stretches, and soft tissue work, and by performing lots of strength exercises designed to restore balance to your body. Most lifters, assuming they even know about such techniques, consider them "small stuff" that they hastily skip over on their way to the bench. And then they wonder why their shoulders are in constant pain, their back gives out, they can barely get out of bed in the morning, and they stop making any progress in the gym. Many of the most successful lifters have said that they attribute their success to staying healthy. It's much easier to do a 10-minute foam-rolling and mobility session at the beginning of each training session than it is to go through 6 to 12 months of rehabilitation for a serious injury.

By now I hope and trust that you see just how big the benefits of such small stuff are. Keep doing it as long as you keep lifting.

MIX UP YOUR EXERCISES

Variety is a major feature of the Maximum Strength Program and should remain a major feature of your training regimen in the future. You performed more than 70 different strength movements in my 16-week program. Sure, some of them were quite similar to one another, but even small variations make a difference. Including a wide range of exercises in your strength training is important for two main reasons. First, it is necessary to achieve a balanced musculoskeletal system, which is the foundation for strength performance. The body is capable of moving in a huge number of different ways. If your gym routine covers only a small fraction of these possible movements, you cannot achieve muscle balance. You must consistently hit all four corners of the map of possible strength movements to achieve adequate balance.

Movement variation is also a variable that can stimulate strength gains directly when manipulated properly alongside other variables, including load and volume. Certain exercises serve as support movements for other exercises. For example, in this program you did side bridges, Pallof presses, and suitcase deadlifts before you attempted any rotational training. Those initial movements prepared your body to rotate properly when you did rotate. Doing the right support movement at the right time can strengthen a muscle or movement pattern that is currently limiting your performance in another exercise. In other words, exercise variation is a valuable tool to eliminate weak links.

The more experienced you become in strength training, the more you will need to vary your exercise selection to stimulate further gains. When you walk into the gym for the first time, just about anything you do will make you stronger. If all you've been doing before then is sitting on the couch, bench pressing will actually make your legs stronger. But the further you go along the path toward your genetic strength limit, the harder it becomes to keep the momentum going. Only unaccustomed training stimuli (greater loads, higher volume, new movements, etc.) can stimulate positive adaptations, and after 10 years of consistent training, your muscles start to think they're accustomed to everything. Throwing in new movements—not just any old exercises, but new movements with a purpose—is a great way to convince your muscles otherwise. A great example would be the inclusion of some Lynx grips (www.lynxpt.com), which serve to make the barbell slightly thicker. It's variation, not a complete change, but your system will respond well to the subtle modification.

There are a lot of strength exercises out there. Keep a lookout for unfamiliar exercises that seem to be worth trying, and try them.

PULL MORE THAN YOU PUSH

You might have noticed that—in sharp contrast to the way most people train in the gym—the Maximum Strength Program includes more pulling exercises than pushing exercises. This pattern is no accident. Primarily because of the tremendous amounts of sitting involved in the modern lifestyle, our pulling muscles tend to be weaker than our pushing muscles. Almost everyone in today's society exhibits this imbalance by adolescence, but weightlifters make it worse by training their pushing muscles more than their pulling muscles.

To develop the balance of strength that is needed to maximize your overall strength, you need to do just the opposite: Pull (i.e., perform rows, deadlifts, pull-ups) more than you push. The Maximum Strength Program has gotten you started in the right direction. Now it's up to you to continue.

DO SINGLE-LEG WORK

One of the most pervasive specific flaws in typical strength-training programs is inadequate use of single-leg movements such as lunges. Such movements are critical tools in maximizing performance in single-leg movements themselves and in double-leg movements such as the deadlift and box squat. Single-leg movements challenge muscles that are not much challenged by double-leg movements and therefore tend to become weak links in those who seldom perform exercises featuring alternating leg actions.

Single-leg movements are also much more specific to most sports activities than double-leg movements. If you do any sport that involves running, for example, then single-leg movements are an essential part of your strength training for that sport.

As I'm sure you recall, single-leg movements are a big part of the Maximum Strength Program. Be sure they remain a big part of your future training.

VARY YOUR TRAINING STRESS

Typical strength-training programs also suffer from inadequate workload modulation. (Workload equals the volume of training times the average intensity of training.) Most guys lift moderately hard every single week. This is not a good recipe for rapid progress. Improvement occurs much more quickly and steadily when heavy-training weeks are alternated with lighter weeks. The heavier weeks slightly overwhelm the body, creating a strong stimulus for adaptation. The lighter weeks provide an opportunity for those adaptations to unfold.

I should make it very clear that when I say "hard," I'm not just referring to *heavy*. Rather, *hard* refers to the overall stress you place on your body. This might be a function of total volume (sets times reps times load), exercise selection (e.g., a deadlift is harder than a leg curl), training frequency (days per week), or any of a number of other factors. Training (1) heavier, (2) with more volume, (3) with more challenging exercises, and (4) with greater frequency will require you to take a step back and rest more often.

The Maximum Strength Program features a four-week workload modulation pattern in which the first week is heavy, the second week is moderate, the third week is very heavy, and the fourth week is light. I have found that this pattern works extremely well for the majority of recreational weightlifters. Feel free to play around with it in the future, but always vary your training stress in a controlled and sensible manner. Don't go back to being a "Johnny One-Note" in your training workload.

KEEP LEARNING AND ADAPTING

As I have implied in making some of my previous points in this chapter, I do encourage ongoing experimentation and experience-based refinement in one's training. I would never suggest that the Maximum Strength Program is the perfect, one-size-fits-all program for every lifter, down to its last detail. There is no single training program that's perfect for everyone. In fact, there's no single training program that's perfect for *anyone*, because each of our bodies is constantly changing. Indeed, the best training programs change our bodies the most, requiring us to make the most changes in our future training to keep the momentum going.

To maximize your long-term gains in the gym, you have to pay attention constantly to how your body responds to various training patterns and use this information to improve your training bit by bit as you go. Some lifters can handle more volume than others. Some lifters need more mobility work than others. Some lifters recover faster than others. To give you one specific personal example, I have found that my body needs and benefits from greater amounts of single-leg work than some other powerlifters need—so I do more. The examples are endless. Observe yourself closely to see what you seem to need, and tweak your training accordingly.

ADJUST YOUR ENERGY
WORKOUTS AS NECESSARY

Energy workouts are an optional component of the Maximum Strength Program, because the program is focused on the objective of building strength, whereas energy workouts are most useful to achieve the objectives of optimizing body composition and improving health. Because these are worthy objectives, I encourage everyone who follows the Maximum Strength Program to follow the somatotype-specific energy workout guidelines I provided, and I hope you did so.

Depending on the results you achieved using these guidelines and your future goals for body composition and health, you may wish to modify your energy workouts going forward. For example, if you made a fairly significant commitment to energy workouts during the 16-week Maximum Strength Program and you feel this commitment limited your strength gains, you might choose to back off the cardio somewhat in the future and rely more on careful eating to stay lean. If, however, you took a minimalist approach to energy workouts and did not lose as much body fat as you hoped to lose, you might choose to make a greater commitment to energy workouts in the future. Training-program design will always involve give and take among competing goals, so it takes time and experimentation to find the right fit for you.

REFINE YOUR
NUTRITION

By continually modifying your training based on self-observation, you will make more progress in the future than you would make if you continued to train exactly the same way you trained during the Maximum Strength Program. The same rule applies to nutrition. The Precision Nutrition guidelines I provided in Chapter 10 establish the optimal framework for a lifetime of healthy eating for maximum performance. But they are general guidelines and leave plenty of room for individual variation in their application.

As with training refinements, finding the best way to apply the Precision Nutrition guidelines to your diet requires ongoing self-observation. Always keep an eye out for problems or limitations that you encounter in your quest for greater health and performance that might have a nutritional origin, and make any necessary adjustments. For example, you might notice that you feel sluggish after eating even the limited amount of grain-based food that the Precision Nutrition guidelines allow, and therefore choose to reduce your intake of such foods even further.

Diet is complex, and it is not always easy to discern when a problem or limitation has a nutritional origin, or to identify the specific origins. Nevertheless, you will be better off making the effort to refine your diet continually to better suit your needs than to just live with the problems and limitations you experience.

APPENDIX

For more information on Eric Cressey's Maximum Strength Program, visit www.EricCressey.com.

Special Bonus Page for Maximum Strength Readers:
http://www.ericcressey.com/maxstrength.html

These Online Bonuses include:
1. Recommended Further Reading
2. Complementary Products
3. Exercise Demonstration Videos from the Maximum Strength Text
4. *Free* Weekly Newsletter
5. *Free* Expert Tip Downloads
6. Maximum Strength Blog with Q&A, Supplemental Information, and Training Videos

Other Products Available from Eric Cressey:

- Magnificent Mobility DVD (www.MagnificentMobility.com)
- Building the Efficient Athlete DVD Set
  (www.BuildingtheEfficientAthlete.com)
- The Ultimate Off-Season Training Manual
  (www.UltimateOffSeason.com)

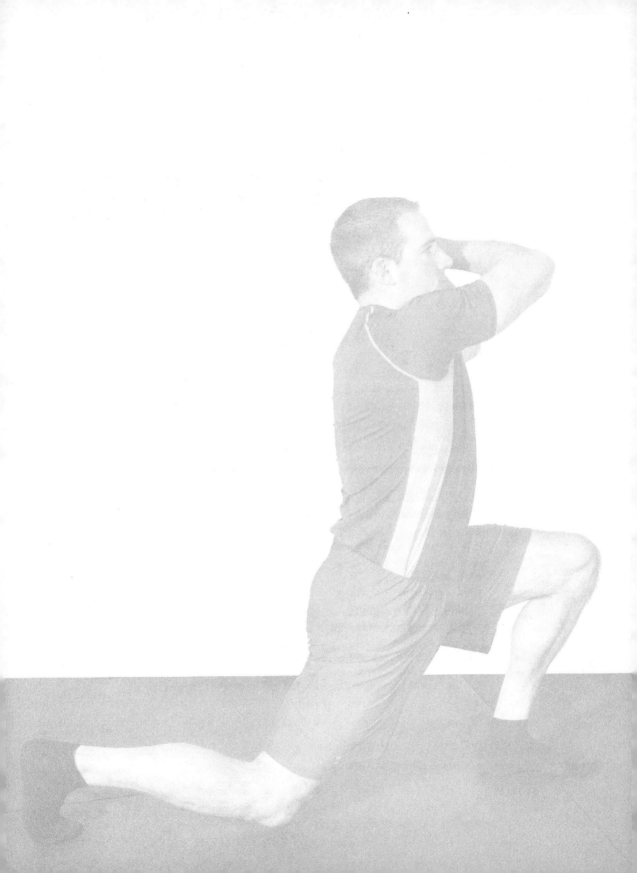

ACKNOWLEDGMENTS

Eric Cressey and Matt Fitzgerald wish to thank the following individuals whose invaluable help made this book possible, and better than it would have otherwise been: John Berardi, PhD; Alwyn Cosgrove; Peter Dupuis; Nataki Fitzgerald; Tony Gentilcore; Audrey Hall; Bill Hartman; David Jenkins; Linda Konner; William Kraemer, PhD; Tim Noakes, MD; Cindy Pitts; Mike Robertson; Renée Sedliar; Anna Sleeper; and all of the athletes and clients—both past and present—who have made us what we are today.

INDEX